Surviving the Zombie Apocalypse

First Aid Kit Building and Mini Med School for Preppers

Dr. Ryan Chamberlin
THEPREPPERPAGES.COM

TABLE OF CONTENTS

iv

WHO ARE WE?

ThePrepperPages.com is a group of physicians who've spent cumulative lifetimes responding to medical misadventures which ultimately led to the writing of this book. In the past medical knowledge has been kept from those who are not part of the sacred healthcare club. We're trying to remedy some of that with the penning of this guide.

The medical profession would have you believe only those initiated by a lifetime of schooling are qualified to provide health care. This isn't true. Army medics, paramedics and navy corpsman are well trained in short periods of time. This is true for zombie preppers, the specialists of self-sufficiency and self-education. For these souls the information age has come along and leveled the playing field. Limits to education and barriers to experience have fallen away before them.

Zombie Apocalypse is designed to teach you how to think through the treatment of trauma and illness. If you're without supplies, you'll learn how to make and collect the tools you'll need while navigating to safety.

The manual is a compilation and revision of our three previous works. Some subjects have been removed, while others have been added.

Dividing into four sections, the book begins with first aid kit construction integrated with easy to perform procedures not found elsewhere. Our second section tackles pandemics and setting up aid stations for treating people without getting ill yourself. The third focuses on pulmonary diseases like pneumonia and lung collapse. This section is important because they've been shown to be prevalent during disasters. Last, we address mental preparedness and the treatment of anxiety and depression. Both bound to be plentiful at the world's end.

Thank you for purchasing this book. We guarantee to teach you more than you've probably ever learned elsewhere!

How to Use this Book

Since we first published The Prepper Pages in 2012, the way digital books like Kindle render images has changed little.   It's still "sub-optimal."

To remedy this we've hyperlinked tables, videos and diagrams to our gallery at Zombie Apocalypse Book Images. If you are viewing this on a digital reader click on the image to enlarge.   Our paperback readers can visit our images page and find them in the order they appear in the book.

The Prepper Page's YouTube Channel supports this guide with instructional videos we've made on suturing, injecting anesthetics, and other helpful procedures.

Our blog can be found in two places: our site under "New Posts," and at blogger Survival Medicine - ThePrepperPages.com.   You can subscribe to either, but we usually post on our site first.

Finally, if you have any questions you can contact us by email or through our contact us page.   Please like us on Facebook and follow us on Twitter!

Is THERE REALLY GOING TO BE A ZOMBIE APOCALYPSE?

Non-preppers rarely miss the opportunity for a dramatic eye roll at the mention of a zombie apocalypse. They view it as a silly but toxic craze polluting popular culture, hoping it will soon fade away like bell bottom jeans and Valley Girls.

Many don't realize it's often a metaphor, and society is in the process of doing what it always has. It's creating a modern day myth; a type of public dream the late mythologist Joseph Campbell was famous for dissecting.

If alive today he might say the story of a zombie virus is the reflection of a fear burrowed deep within the human psyche. Generational memory of the terror experienced during a predictable event called plague - a true story playing out for centuries. He might even add people have been expressing their anxieties in this form since the beginning of the written word. Stories like these are designed to protect our sanity by presenting danger in a light-hearted way.

Of course there's always the possibility some type of zombie virus really is hidden behind some squirmy little lab nerd; both coiled and waiting to pounce. Perhaps it's something we haven't seen yet.   In the era of genetically modified everything... *who knows what to expect?*

The Zombie Virus - in whichever form it takes - is likely to become a pandemic because many countries don't have the soap and water necessary for their people to keep clean.   If they do, some can't maintain their borders or prevent egress of the ill without their militaries springing into genocide mode.   These places represent a clear danger to The United States of America and her allies.

Pandemics have destabilized countless armies and nations throughout history.   Back then our connection to one another was spotty.   Separated by impassable mountain ranges and angry seas, the isolation slowed and often stopped rampaging diseases.   That protection no longer exists.   Nowadays we must expect geometric growth in infection rates.   The epicenters of the next zombie virus will likely be in third world slum-cities.   The disease reaching outward from there, we can subsequently expect entire countries to collapse.   And when that mass builds to critical, the dominoes falling will be continents, one burning after the other.   Destruction will continue until its fuel has been exhausted, and then we'll have more zombies than trees in our backyards.

Many people don't realize the Central Intelligence Agency has a medical division for monitoring illness in each region of the world.   A section that trying to predict the way public health concerns might reshape the political and military geography of the world.   They've created and maintained this division because they know it's a serious threat in our modern world; no matter how far away the problem might be centered.

In under a month Ebola exposed America's weak spots. But it also bought us some breathing room for making preparations. If it had been as contagious as influenza we'd never learned what we have. Now we can prepare for the next virus, or for the arrival of one of its friends who's reactivated in a remote jungle reservoir.

The flu of 1918 killed millions here. At that time the world's population was less than a third it is now. That was fortunate because it meant there were far fewer people which could transmit the disease. The virus eventually burned itself out, as people of the time lived mostly in rural and isolated communities.

But those places no longer exist. The interconnected nature of humanity has unintentionally dismantled the best safety valve protecting us from epidemics. We've lost one of our most important tools - *and we'll never get it back.*

SECTION ONE

SCAVENGING YOUR KIT & PUTTING IT TO USE WHILE FLEEING FROM THE UNDEAD

GETTING YOUR BEARINGS

Throughout this book are "text boxes" This type box contains vital points and things to remember.

Items to Collect While Bugging Out

THESE BOXES TELL YOU WHAT TO LOOK FOR (WHAT TO "BORROW") AS YOU SEARCH A HOUSE OR LOOTED STORE, WHILE ON YOUR DASH TO SAFETY.

It used to be hard to find medical equipment. Those days are gone. You don't need a medical license to order most supplies anymore; particularly when buying them from overseas. The Internet gives zombie preppers access to almost anything, including supplies once limited only to physicians.

The only disclaimer we will make is that if professional medical care is available, or will be available, then always use it. Follow a doctor's treatment and advice. No one is advocating the practice of medicine without a license, or breaking into a pharmacy without a life threatening emergency. That being said, this book is written for when society and its conveniences fall away. As you know with catastrophes, conventional medical care is seldom available. This puts the medical care of your family and friends on you.

Medications and Special Instructions

The particulars of key medications and specialized instructions for procedures are summarized here.

More detailed information will often be included in the appendices.

You'll see text boxes scattered throughout these pages. Some contain important tips, others specific directions. Capitalized boxes are designed to convey motion. The kind you're engaged in when rifling through the rooms of a house, or the shelves of a looted store while on your way to safety.

During hurricane Katrina it took 78 hours before the veneer of humanity fell away. In the first 48 hours people helped one another. Two days later they were stealing from the same people they first helped. Their behavior was bizarre, and later reminded many of the book Lord of the Flies. In later television interviews, it became clear just how easily people justified their insane actions.

Many said they had to do whatever was necessary to take care of their families. While their duty was understandable, their escapades often went far beyond that needed. "Greed is good" once again guided the hearts of man. The separation between human and pack animal narrowed. Most expected more out of Americans, and most were profoundly disappointed. We need to expect history is again about to repeat itself.

<u>Side Notes</u>: These Sections Provide More Information About Important Topics in the Chapter.

Now let's get to the action!

BAGGING TREASURES

Say civilization has been wrestled face down. That order is loosely controlled, and even then only by the tightest of force. What would happen to people with valued skills? Would they be safe? Would their children be free?

In dark times identifying yourself as having medical skills or equipment might be fatal. People with special abilities have often been kidnapped for their talents. This happened to an American friend of ours while on vacation overseas. On his first night in the country, a military coup rudely woke him. He was an Orthopedic Surgeon, and found himself conscripted into the country's new provisional army.

Weeks went by before realizing if he was ever to leave, he would have to go to the warlord and plead for release. He knew his request could get him killed. But he got lucky. The commander thanked him for his service and allowed him to leave. But it could have gone south.

> Put your medical kit in a plain unmarked bag. Be careful not to let anyone know you have skills or supplies.

The story is told of a well-known news correspondent who had a similar experience in 1991, back when the Military first went into Iraq.   He was there covering the story when a ranking officer learned he was a neurosurgeon before becoming a reporter.   His microphone was taken away and replaced with surgical scrubs.   He was pointed to the operating room and put to work.

Water Proofing

In the kitchen you'll find thick black trash and Ziploc bags. Grab several trash bags, reinforcing one inside the other. Stuff all the items you're collecting into these bags. Keep moving!

It's said that he was there for two weeks before his news agency was able to liberate him from Iraq.   If the United States Military could do this, imagine what a misguided militia group would be capable of if they find you with special skills or equipment. Sometimes it's better to be ordinary, or at least convey that impression.

When you buy a medical kit, keep it in an unmarked and plain looking bag. You wouldn't want to get shot for your supplies. Put it into something non-assuming to avoid curious eyes.

Never forget to put your supplies and equipment into individually sealed plastic or Ziploc bags. The items in your kit must remain waterproof at all times!

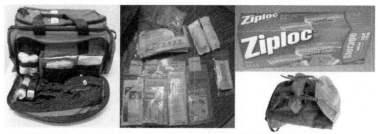

PUT YOUR MEDICAL SUPPLIES INTO A LESS OBVIOUS BAG THAN THE ONE SHOWN ON THE LEFT. PLACE EVERYTHING INTO HEAVY SEALABLE STORAGE BAGS (CENTER). IT'S BEST TO PUT YOUR KIT INTO AN OLD SURPLUS BAG LIKE THE ONE ON THE RIGHT.

It's important to keep your kit as small as possible. After assembling your medical supplies, you'll want to save most of the rest of the room in your pack for water, food and specialized clothing. Water creates a unique problem because it weighs eight pounds a gallon, and takes up a lot of space. But at the same time, it's the most essential element of life.

Later on we'll talk about making water potable. Improvising a water filter can minimize what you need to carry. But if there's no water in the environment, there's nothing to filter. This is something to consider if you have to travel through dry environments. In the swamps of Florida, this isn't such a concern.

Coffee Filters

WHILE MOVING THROUGH THE KITCHEN COLLECT AND "POCKET" SOME COFFEE FILTERS. NEXT LOOK AT THE SINK FAUCET. IF YOU SEE AN AFTERMARKET WATER FILTER, DETACH IT AND PUT IT IN YOUR BAG. THE COFFEE FILTERS CAN BE USED TO SIEVE PARTICULATE MATTER OUT OF DIRTY WATER, AND PARTS FROM THE FAUCET FILTER CAN BE USED LATER TO BUILD A QUALITY FILTER FOR DRINKING & MEDICAL USE.

For now let's move on to talk about bandages. When we do, we are referring to wound dressings or coverings and not standard Band-Aids.

Gauze dressings take up a lot of space. Almost everyone packs too few... *or way too many.* You only need a small number, but the ones you have should be individually wrapped and sterile. That's because these will be the dressings coming in direct contact with fresh wounds. If not sterile, they become potential sources of infection.

Square shaped bandages are usually made of weaved and scratchy gauze. They're sold in two and four inch squares, called two by two's, and four by four's respectively.

If you buy the unwrapped type, they'll come in a brick like bundle. You can get a lot of them cheaply this way, but remember they aren't sterile - only clean. And that's alright for many purposes, but for fresh cuts you'll need the individually wrapped sterile units.

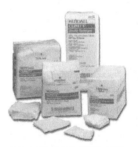 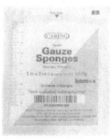 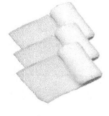

INDIVIDUALLY WRAPPED AND BULK GAUZE. BULK ARE STERILE ONLY IF THE PACKAGE IS UNOPENED

COME IN TWO SIZES 4X4, AND 2X2 INCHES - FOR DIRECT CONTACT WITH SKIN

ROLLED GAUZE CAN BE WRAPPED AROUND A LIMB

It's best to carry a few 4x4s individually packaged and sterile for placing over new wounds, then plan on reinforcing them with non-sterile or even makeshift dressings. That way you'll only need a few sterile gauze in your kit. One or two of these, held in place by a bed sheet or pillow case you've scavenged, can save lots of space.

Sterile dressings can be difficult to find as they're rarely left behind after looting. But you can use almost anything as a bandage. Just make sure it's clean. In WWII, Catholic nuns acting as combat nurses used cut up bed sheets and strips of mattress for dressings. They found that as long as they were relatively clean, they worked well. Keep this trick in mind.

Pillow Cases & Linens

LOOK IN THE LINEN CLOSET. GRAB PLAIN WHITE PILLOW CASES AND STUFF THEM INTO YOUR BAG, OR USE THEM AS A BAG IF YOU DON'T HAVE ONE. THEY CAN BE CUT INTO STRIPS, ROLLED UP, AND USED FOR DRESSINGS AND SLINGS LATER. NOW GO INTO THE BATHROOM AND FIND A JAR OF VASELINE, AND ANY MEDICAL SUPPLIES YOU CAN FIND. PUT THEM IN YOUR BAG AND KEEP MOVING!

Along with sterile dressings, buy or find individual packets of antibacterial ointment and Vaseline. You rarely need a whole tube or jar, unless that's all that's available. Small packets of antibiotic ointment take up little room, and can be used to coat the contacting surface of the dressing. This is a way of creating an inexpensive non-adhering wound cover. If the dressing doesn't stick, it won't be painful when you have to change it.

Bandages should be changed every 24 hours, unless they soak through sooner. In that case change them as needed. Wounds heal best when slightly moist, not completely dry. This is another good reason to use antibiotic ointment or Vaseline. Dry and uncovered wounds were once thought to heal faster, but this has been disproven in several recent studies.

As a general rule, simple lacerations take 24 hours to seal over. The dressing's inner surface only needs to be sterile until then. After that, it just needs to be clean. Once sealed shut the injury is unlikely to become infected from an unsterile gauze.

If it does become infected, it's usually because the wound couldn't be irrigated well when initially cleaned and dressed; or because small foreign bodies harboring bacteria were missed during the process.

When it comes to dressings, sometimes people get crazy. I remember a patient that had an abdominal operation a week before, leaving him with a large but healing incision. After the seventh day he ran out of fresh bandages and decided to improvise. He found an old sock and a roll of duct tape. But the sock was filthy. "No problem" he reasoned, and fixed that by soaking it in gasoline... then he duct taped it on. The resulting skin burn and allergic reaction were impressive. Improvisation is good, but too much can be bad.

ACE™ or elastic bandages have many valuable uses. But for single use there's something even better. Often referred to by its trade name 3M Vetrap, it's a dressing that looks like an Ace, but sticks to itself. It's stretchy and doesn't need to be cut. You can tear it like masking tape.

Veterinarians use it on animals because it stays on better than elastic bandages. It comes in two, four, and six inch widths. One roll can be used many times because you never end up needing the whole thing. But once applied, that section cannot be used again after being removed.

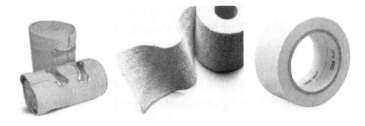

ACE BANDAGES (LEFT) ARE ELASTIC AS IS "VET TAPE" (MIDDLE)
BOTH CAN BE WRAPPED AROUND A LIMB WITHOUT RISKING
CUTTING OFF THE BLOOD SUPPLY. NON-ELASTIC TAPE (RIGHT)
CANNOT. IT MUST BE TORN INTO STRIPS FIRST.

Once you've selected your bandages, there's one other important consideration. While more expensive, some dressings come impregnated with antibiotics or other ointments. You place them in-between the wound and gauze to prevent the two from adhering. They may also help in preventing infections. Known best by the trade names Adaptic and Xeroform, you can find similar products that are generic and cheaper. If you're putting together a well-stocked medical bag, you'll want a few.

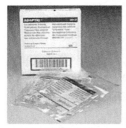
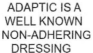
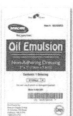

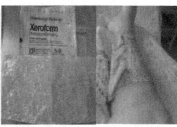

ADAPTIC IS A WELL KNOWN NON-ADHERING DRESSING	OIL EMULSION AND XEROFORM DRESSINGS ARE ALSO WIDELY USED	DRESSING CHANGES ARE EASIER WITH NON-ADHERING

One final word of bandages.   If you're building a kit, try to find a few eye patches.   Most grocery stores carry them.   They're made from a non-abrasive oval shaped gauze called Telfa, another non-adhering dressing.   But it's dry, not moist like those impregnated with ointment.

If you don't have any patches, just cut a 4x4 into an oval shape.   They help stop the pain of pink eye and other infections.   Have the person close their eye, and place a patch over it.   In 24 hours many eye abrasions will heal if covered.   And within two days most ocular infections will resolve.   Eye injuries and infections are usually minor. Though most people don't think so because they really hurt. More on their treatment later in the book.

Now let's see what you'll really need; what you must have to live.

SHANKING - SCALPELS & BOX CUTTERS

Rule 9- "Never go anywhere without a knife"
- Leroy Jethro Gibbs, NCIS

Some of the best places to order materials are from companies catering to veterinarians. Many operate outside the country, and most are accessible online. The secret here is that they have the same instruments and supplies used for humans, though they don't advertise it for legal reasons. Many items are up to 80% less expensive when purchased this way, and most companies don't require any sort of medical license. Amazon is another great resource, but items there are often more expensive.

One of the first things you'll need is a scalpel, or a small sharp knife. Preferably you'll have already purchased scalpels. If not you can often find a box cutter, X-ACTO® or sheetrock knife. These can work like a #11 blade scalpel, one of the most useful types for field work.

Improvised Scalpels

MAKE YOUR WAY TO THE GARAGE. LOOK FOR DUCT TAPE AND BOX CUTTERS OR SHEETROCK KNIVES. IF YOU CAN'T FIND A BLADE, MAKE YOUR WAY TO THE KIDS' ROOMS. THEY MAY HAVE AN X-ACTO® KNIFE IN THEIR ARTS AND CRAFT SUPPLIES. IF THE KIDS ARE OLDER, THEY MAY ALSO HAVE SOME "HERBAL REMEDIES" HIDDEN, THEY CAN BE USED FOR PAIN CONTROL LATER.

For the purposes of a medical kit there're two types of scalpels, disposable and non-disposable. With the non-disposable or reusable, you have to replace the blade and sterilize the handle after each use. Using this setup can save a little room in your kit, because you only need one handle for use with many small and tightly packaged blades. Each small blade is discarded after use. But you have to sterilize the handle every time you use it. Problems can arise at times, because some blades don't fit all handles.

Disposable scalpels come with the blade already attached, but take up a little more room. I prefer these. I've even used them in the operating room. This is because many have a retractable sheath, which has prevented me from accidently stabbing myself or my justifiably nervous assistants.   With the reusable types I've cut myself a few times trying to place the scalpel blade onto the handle.

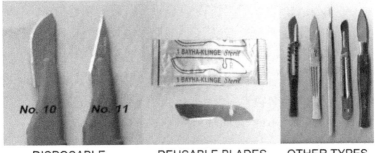

| DISPOSABLE SCALPELS | REUSABLE BLADES NEEDING A STERILE HANDLE | OTHER TYPES YOU MAY SEE |

All disposable equipment, regardless if it's a scalpel, suture, needle, or syringe, should be discarded after use. But sometimes this isn't practical.   Especially when you know you won't be resupplied in the foreseeable future.

If you do recycle your disposables, mark them as such, and disinfect them as best possible.   But do so knowing no matter how good the cleaning job, they're still capable of transmitting disease.   This is particularly true if they've been contaminated by infected blood or secretions.

That being said, contracting a communicable disease from a used blade or needle will probably be the least of your problems in an era when zombies are continually getting caught up in your truck's axel.   We'll discuss how to sterilize equipment in the field and taking precautions against infection a bit later in the book.

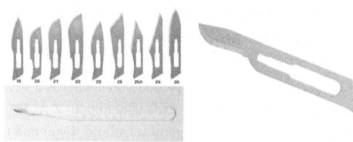

SCALPELS ARE NAMED BY NUMBER (LEFT TOP)
#15 BLADES ARE THE MOST USEFUL FOR FIELD
PURPOSES (LEFT BOTTOM and RIGHT)

Scalpels are classified strangely. They're named by a number that indicates their shape. The shape of each type of blade serves a particular purpose. Some can be used for multiple tasks.

A #15 blade will do just about everything you need. If you buy only one scalpel make it a #15. It's great for cutting away dead skin before suturing, a procedure called debridement, and a variety of other creative uses.

Next time you are at your doctor's office, ask if you could have a scalpel or two for your emergency kit. If you're buying scalpels, they come 10 to a box, all of which are the same shape. Get #15 blades in this case.

If you can get two, the second you'll want is a #11 blade. These are shaped like a triangle, and an X-ACTO® knife or box cutter works as a good substitute if you don't have your kit. They can usually be found in the junk drawers of most kitchens, or the garages of most homes.

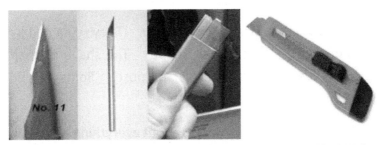

X-Acto KNIFES AND BOX CUTTERS CAN BE EASILY FOUND WHEN YOU ARE ON THE MOVE - THEY MAKE GOOD SUBSTITUTES FOR #11 SCALPELS

Triangular blades are excellent for draining abscesses, a common ailment in disaster zones. For now, know that the triangular # 11 blade, or its equivalent, will be one of the most useful tools in your aid kit.

24

That's really all that you need to know about scalpels. There will be more detailed information when we discuss suturing and wound care. Be sure to cover the blade in some way after use. And remember that even disposable scalpels will keep their edge over long periods of time. They can probably be used five times for delicate work, and another 10 for general use... if necessary.

Batteries & Remotes

IN TRANSIT BETWEEN THE ROOMS OF A HOME, PAUSE IN THE FAMILY AND LIVING ROOMS, AND LOOK FOR A SCRAP BOOK. AN X-ACTO KNIFE MAY BE NEAR BY. NEXT, STRIP ALL OF THE BATTERIES OUT OF THE GAMING CONTROLLERS AND TV REMOTES. TOSS THEM INTO YOUR BAG AND KEEP MOVING.

One thing never to be disposed of in the field, not when you're sure you'll never be resupplied... is your gloves.

They are second only to your knife!

GLOVING UP AND CUTTING DOWN

Rule 2- *"Always wear gloves at a crime scene"*
- Leroy Jethro Gibbs, NCIS

Gloves protect you, and that's always first! The real purpose of gloves, is to protect you from getting whatever the person you are working on might have. In the field, gloves are likely to be cleaner than your hands. With that in mind, remember that one of the most important things you can have in your bag is soap. Non-scented antibacterial is best.

Soap

RIFLE THROUGH THE BATHROOM. FIND A BAR OF SOAP AND DROP IT IN YOUR BAG. NEXT TIME YOU OR A FRIEND ARE AT A HOTEL, SWIPE THE SMALL BARS OF SOAP AND PUT THEM IN YOUR AID KIT.

In the environments we are functioning in you'll want to be clean - *but not smell clean.* Soap perfume can be detected from surprising distances and can draw the same level of attention as grilling steak. But it's every bit as valuable to your health as antibiotics, and the one thing many forget to pack.

Carry bar soap only, it can always be made into a liquid solution later. Remember that even when the soap is antibacterial, it only helps make your hands cleaner, not sterile or even well sanitized.

Vegitable Peelers & Dishwashing

WHEN IN THE KITCHEN LOOK UNDER THE SINK. GRAB THOSE HEAVY LONG SLEEVED GLOVES USED FOR WASHING DISHES. THEY'RE A GREAT SUBSTITUTE IF YOU DON'T HAVE YOUR EXAM GLOVES OR KIT WITH YOU. FIND A VEGITABLE PEELER, THEN GRAB A KITCHEN SPONGE.
YOU CAN USE THE SPONGE FOR FILTERING WATER BEFORE PURIFICATION, AND THE PEELER FOR MAKING SOAP SHAVINGS.

The gloves you use are just as important as having them. But the way they function is poorly understood and deliberately deceptive.

Consider the people working in drive-thru windows or cash registers. You'll often see them wearing clear vinyl gloves.

They're trying to protect themselves from getting the flu or the common cold. Both are caused by viruses that can be carried on money. But while their intention is right, their method is wrong. Vinyl gloves have pores in them much larger than any virus. Wearing them is equivalent to trying to avoid machine gun fire by taking cover behind a chain-link fence - *literally*. The math on the proportions used in this analogy is almost precise.

Vinyl is preferred by employers. It's inexpensive and avoids latex exposure for their employees; many of whom have successfully sued in decades past. But it doesn't protect the worker from viral infections, only some bacterial pathogens.

To protect yourself from viruses you'll need latex or nitrile gloves. Color coded either blue or purple, nitrile gloves have small enough pores to block viral pathogens.

Latex, usually yellow but sometimes green, is also protective. The drawback is the allergy issue. Most hospitals disposed of products made from latex years ago. But latex gloves are still available for Surgeons and in non-hospital settings. Sometimes you'll see police donning them in the background of newscasts. These gloves are generally inexpensive and easy to find.

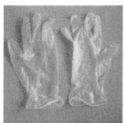 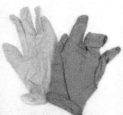 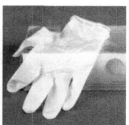

| VINYL GLOVES DO NOT PROTECT YOU FROM VIRUSES LIKE HIV, HEPATITIS, OR EVEN THE FLU | NITRILE GLOVES WERE ORIGINALLY MADE FOR PEOPLE WITH LATEX ALLERGIES | LATEX AND NITRILE ARE THE ONLY COMMON GLOVES THAT PROTECT AGAINST VIRUSES |

Contrast that to surgical gloves, which come sterile and wrapped in pairs. Each package has a very specific size. They're required for sterile procedures and are expensive. If you're going to use these find out what size fits you first. Seven-and- a-half and 8 are typical sizes for most men, 6 ½ to 7 for most women.

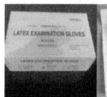 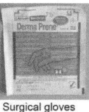 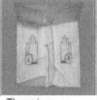

| Non-Sterile box of latex gloves. Usually contain 50 pairs and protect against viral and bacterial pathogens. | Surgical gloves come sterile and in specific sizes. Most packages have right and left gloves, but you must be sure. | There is a specific protocol for removing the gloves from the package in a sterile fashion. | Surgical gloves are sized to fit, so know yours before ordering. These are not typically needed for our purposes. |

Nitrile and non-surgical latex gloves are sold by the box and come in less precise sizes: small, medium, large, and extra-large. Though not sterile, they're worth every inch of space they occupy in your bag.

Side Note: Avoiding Bar Soap & Staying Healthy

Wearing medical gloves all day might keep you from picking up unwanted germs, but's obviously impractical. So we recommend wearing tactical, shooting, or driving gloves regularly.   You can scavenge a pair from an auto parts store or Walmart.   They offer some protection against pathogens commonly contracted when touching contaminated items in the environment.

Doorknobs are the worst in this regard, but just about any other smooth object people frequently touch can do the same.   These surfaces are called fomites in the medical world.   You must aggressively protect yourself against the germs they may be harboring if you're to stay healthy.

Pens and stethoscopes are two of the most common fomites associated with health care providers.   Doctors nowadays often clean their stethoscopes with rubbing alcohol in-between patients.

It seems that by forming biofilms, especially on the surfaces of smooth objects like table tops and drawer handles, infectious organisms can be transferred effortlessly form one person to another.   Three surprising facts have emerged from recent research into this matter.

First, paper money, which was long thought of as a major fomite, does not transfer infection as often as once thought. Porous materials like cloth, which is really what money is printed on, absorbs and traps contagions to some degree, making it more difficult to pass infection through simple contact.

Second, the five second rule for eating food you've dropped turns out to be valid. I've no idea how researches managed to secure a grant for that study, but they did.

Third, bar soap, in being smooth and coming into contact with multiple people, confers a high transmission rate. Yes, you can get sick from soap, *even if it's antibacterial.* This presents an obvious paradox. Because frequent hand washing is one of best defenses against contagious illness. So what's the solution? If you've run out of Purell, then it's time to make soap shavings.

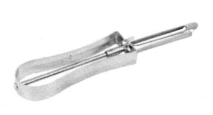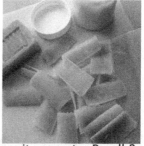

Bar soap can transmit as many illnesses as it prevents. Purell & other hand sanitizers avoid this problem, but might be in limited supply. So use a vegetable peeler to make bar soap shavings.

With your vegetable peeler and a brand new bar of soap, peel large strips off and divvy them up amongst your group.   Let them known they're to be used once per hand washing, and to no longer share bar soap.

Now that you have gloves and soap, and are ready to fish around in fresh wounds, let's talk about sewing your friends back together!

STITCHING UP SORROWS - SUTURES & SUTURE MATERIAL

It's like sewing clothes and tying fly fishing knots melted together. "Suture" refers to the type of surgical thread used to repair lacerations. Typically this material will react little with a person's body. But in certain instances, the reaction can be intense. There are hundreds of different types of suture. Choosing the right kind can be confusing.

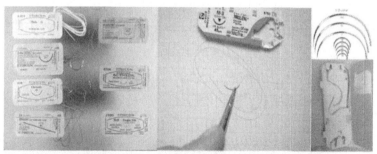

(LEFT) - VARIOUS TYPES AND SIZES OF SUTURES. NOTE THE STRAIT SUTURE NEEDLE ON THE BOTTOM LEFT, AND THE VARIETY OF CURVED NEEDLES IN THE UPPER RIGHT CORNER

Suture comes in many varieties. Absorbable and non-absorbable, braided and non-braided, and even some that have been pre-treated with antibiotics. Suture is rated like fishing line. But instead of "pound-test," a numbering system of zeros "0" is used. The more zeros, the smaller the diameter of the material.

For example, the abbreviation "5-0" means 00000. A package of suture may be marked as 3-0 (000), 6-0 (000000), or any variety of other numbers.

The more zeros, the more delicate the suture. 6-0 suture for instance, is very small, and used for cuts on the face and in other plastic surgeries. This size isn't used often by zombie preppers, a package or two is all most will ever need.

Improvising Suturing Materials

WHILE IN THE GARAGE, LOOK FOR A FISHING TACKLE BOX. TAKE THE CLEAN UNUSED FISHING LINE, NEEDLE NOSE PLIERS (FISHERMEN USE THESE TO REMOVE HOOKS), AND ANY NEEDLES AND SYRINGES YOU FIND (USED BY FISHERMEN TO PUFF UP WORMS WITH AIR.) ALSO GRAB A FEW HOOKS AND LEAD SINKERS FOR FISHING LATER. YOU MIGHT ALSO FIND HAND SANITIZERS LIKE PURELL, THAT'S LIKE DISCOVERING GOLD! NOW KEEP MOVING!

You'll want suture a bit thicker than the thread you'd use to sew clothes. Keep in mind that suture material is designed to be stronger than sewing thread the same size, just as fishing line is. This means that unused or sterilized fishing line can be an acceptable substitute for suture when there's nothing better available. The problem, as you'll remember from fishing, is the material is hard to tie into tight knots. So if you use it to stitch someone back together, tie lots of knots and leave long tails on the ends. Otherwise it can unravel and cause the wound to reopen.

Many of the first modern surgeons had obsessions with fly fishing. Even today their fly knots are taught to surgical residents for using with slippery suture material. It may be easier to use thick sewing thread, and not fishing line, when you're afraid of the knot coming undone.

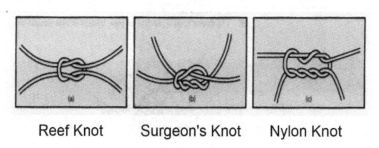

Reef Knot   Surgeon's Knot   Nylon Knot

Here are two videos dealing with tying suture. The first will teach you the easy way by using an instrument, the second by using your hands:

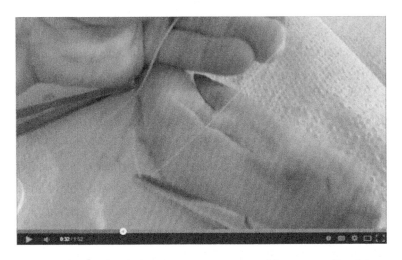

If you don't have an instrument like a needle driver, you can tie it with your hands:

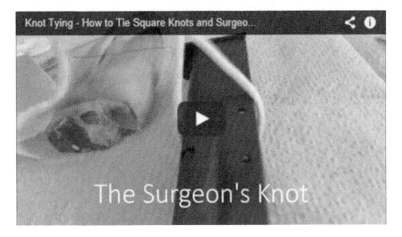

SUTURE SIZES

Most useful are sizes between 2-0 and 5-0. If you can only get one size buy 3-0. It's better to use a heavier material than you need, than selecting a smaller size that might break.

SUTURE SIZES TO USE BY BODY AREA

Suture Sizes by Body Area

Wound location	absorbable	nonabsorbable
Under tension	3-0, 4-0	4-0
Face	5-0	5-0, 6-0
Small or no tension	5-0	5-0
Extremities		4-0, 5-0
Trunk		4-0

Surplus suture can sometimes be bought in bulk from veterinarian suppliers, though in this form only the inside of the package is sterile.   But it's the best way to buy it.   It's inexpensive this way, and comes in a mix of sizes and materials.

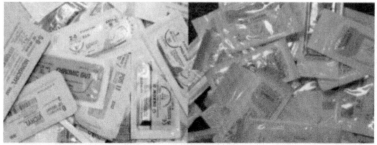

50 piece mixed suture sets available from Amazon.com
Single wrapped packages are shown on the left, double wrapped sterile packages are shown on the right.

> Packages of mixed single wrapped suture materials, and inexpensive surgical instruments, can be found at Amazon.com and other merchants listed in the appendix.

Purchasing suture packaged in a box and wrapped in a second sterile cover can get expensive. Medical students often buy a combination of surplus single packaged units, and use them to practice their surgical technique.

Single packaged material is good enough for most purposes. The material inside is sterile; at least until the package is opened and the suture is removed. I don't use sterile technique in the wilderness any longer. I've found that sterility in the outdoors, and in natural disasters, is wishful thinking at best.

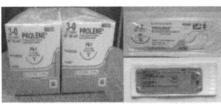
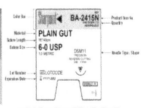

IF YOU BUY SUTURE BY THE BOX, YOU ONLY GET ONE SIZE SUTURE ON ONE SIZE NEEDLE. BUT EACH PACK IS INDIVIDUALLY WRAPPED AND STERILE	SOME TYPES OF SUTURE ARE NO LONGER STERILE AFTER THE OUTER WRAPPING IS REMOVED (TOP) SOME STILL ARE (BOTTOM)	LEARN TO READ THE SUTURE ABBREVIATIONS SHOWN ON THE PACKAGING. OFTEN THE NEEDLE'S PICTURE IS ITS ACTUAL SIZE

Whether you buy a box of sterile suture, or an individual package, the material will usually come attached to a needle. And the needle shown will be its actual size.

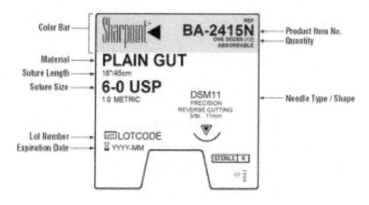

It's best to look at each loose package, ensuring it has a needle pictured before you buy it. That way if you don't need the needle, you can cut it off later. But trying to attach a needle afterword is like trying to herd cats. You end up struggling for hours and wanting to set them on fire.

Suture can be divided into two types, absorbable and non-absorbable. Non-absorbable materials easier to use and more robust. Absorbables are designed for internal use, as with appendectomies or hernia repairs. They can be used to repair skin cuts, but may cause the wound edges to turn red. The resulting discoloration can be mistaken for an infection.

ABSORBABLE MATERIALS

In order to break down and be removed, absorbable suture must activate the immune system. Redness from inflammation, and not necessarily infection, often ensues. So if you use absorbables, expect discoloration and look to other indicators to decide if an infection has developed. Excessive warmth, tenderness, and unclear or foul smelling discharge are signs the repair has gone south.

The names of the older non-synthetic absorbables end with the word "gut." Plain gut and chromic gut being most common. These two materials are known to most people as "cat gut," though they're really made from sterilized sheep intestine. Plain gut sticks around for about a week on the skin before its outer exposed part starts to fall away.

Absorbable Sutures and Their Features			
Product	Features	Advantages	Disadvantages
Gut (plain)	Natural product, absorbed by proteolysis	Inexpensive, maintains tensile strength for 4-5 days	Poor tensile strength, poor knot security, high tissue reactivity, quickly absorbed
Gut (chromic)	Natural product, absorbed by proteolysis	Less tissue reactivity than untreated catgut, prolonged tensile strength	Moderate tissue reactivity, poor knot security
Polyglycolic acid (Dexon)	Synthetic product, monofilament, absorbed by hydrolysis	Delayed absorption, greater tensile and knot strength, diminished tissue reactivity	Stiff, difficult to handle (braided version easier to handle)
Polyglactic acid (Vicryl)	Synthetic product, coated with lubricant, absorbed by hydrolysis	Easy to handle, tensile strength approximately equal to polyglycolic acid, diminished tissue reactivity	Dyed form may be visible through skin
Polyglactic acid (PDS)	Synthetic product, monofilament, hydrolyzes slowly	Extended duration of tensile strength (about 74% at 2 weeks), minimal foreign body reaction	Quite stiff, difficult to handle
Polyglyconate (Maxon)	Synthetic product, monofilament, hydrolyzes slowly	Extended duration of tensile strength (about 81% at 2 weeks), supple, easy to handle	Expensive; new product, limited experience

Plain gut, chromic gut, and Vicryl are the most important absorbable sutures for preppers. Other common forms are also shown, as they may be included in mixed packages of suture, and are very useful to have.

While this means some types of absorbable suture don't need to be removed, it also means they're going to cause inflammation. This can make the wound itch more than usual. Remember that lacerations almost always itch when they're healing, it's a good sign. But excessive pain and tenderness are not.

Characteristics of Absorbable Suture Materials

Material	Tensile strength half-life, days	Tissue reaction	Configuration	Ease of handling	Knot security	Color
Gut (fast absorbing)	2	2	Mono	1	1	N
Gut (plain)	4	4	Mono	1	1	N
Gut (chromic)	7	4	Mono	1	2	N
Dexon	14	2	Braided	3	4	G,W
Vicryl	14	2	Braided	3	4	V, G
PDS	28	2	Mono	2	3	C,V
Maxon	21-28	2	Mono	3	3	C, G

1 – Lowest; 4 - highest

The colors are N=not colored or natural color, G=green, W=white, V=violet, and C=clear. Clear suture can be very difficult to see while sewing, especially at night or in low light.

Chromic gut is also dissolvable, but those stitches have to be removed later. Their chrome coating makes them last longer. Newer synthetic types are made of protein and carbohydrate combinations. They often have the word "glactin" somewhere in their generic name. Vicryl, the brand name for Polyglactin suture, is a common example.

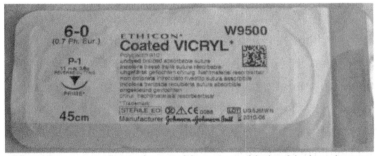

Vicryl is an excellent absorbable suture. It's braided and easy to tie, but must be removed later because it dissolves slowly.

NON-ABSORBABLE MATERIALS

Given the choice, try to stay with non-absorbable materials. They too are made of both natural and artificial fibers. The synthetics are made of nylon or something similar, and like fishing line, can be hard to tie into tight knots.

Some artificial sutures are braided, meaning they have small connected sections along their length. You can feel these tiny indentations by running your fingers down the material. The grooves help lock the suture into place when tied; that's why I recommend braided materials.

The most common and perhaps most useful braided suture is silk. It's cheap and easy to tie with an old fashion square knot. Tie three or four times, cut off the excessive string, and move on to the next one. I carry it in my emergency bag because it's inexpensive and easy to use.

Common Characteristics of Non-Absorbable Suture

Material	Tissue reaction	Configuration	Ease of handling	Knot Security
Silk	4	Braided	4	4
Nylon (mono)	1	Mono	2	2
Nylon (braided)	2	Braided	3	4
Polypropylene	1	Mono	1	1
Polybutester	1	Mono	2	3
Polyester (uncoated)	1	Braided	3	3

1- Lowest; 4 - Highest

It may not surprise you to learn that the first suture was made from cotton, a material that still works well today. It has a higher infection rate than others, but can be found

43

in travel sewing kits. It's not as strong as silk, but that isn't a problem if you use thicker thread, or use two strands at once.

When you're on the move keep an eye out for a sewing kit, it makes a convenient alternative to surgical suture. Moreover, it's likely to be left behind after everything else has been looted from your neighborhood store; and most homes have one. Thread, needles, scissors; all in one compact box.

Sewing Kits & Scissors

LOOK IN THE KITCHEN DRAWERS, COAT CLOSETS, AND DRESSERS FOR A SEWING KIT OR SEWING SUPPLIES. DO THE SAME AS YOU MOVE THROUGH LOOTED STORES. TRAVEL SEWING KITS HAVE EVERYTHING NEEDED FOR IMPROVISED SKIN REPAIRS.

Surgical suturing needles come in many confusing sizes and configurations. Discussed before, suture generally comes with a needle attached. Most needles are curved into a half-circle, others are strait and flat at the end. What's important is that they're labeled "cutting" or "reverse cutting" on the package. Soon we'll cover techniques for suturing. For now just note that most needles are curved. They're shaped this was so that when you stick them in and twist your wrist, they'll naturally travel under the cut and come out on the other side.

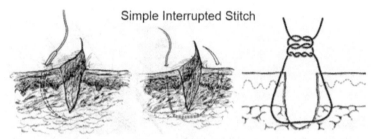

Simple Interrupted Stitch

Curved surgical needles are designed to track underneath the wound and emerge on the other size. You can grab both ends, one in each hand, and tie several square knots. Or you can use an instrument tie to save time.

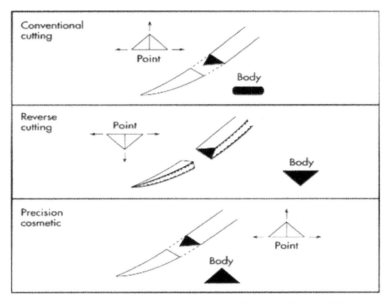

There are many different types of needles, you'll want the kind marked "cutting" or "precision." These usually have one or two letters followed by a number. For instance, FS-2 stands for "For Skin" and has a size 2 needle. PS stands for "Precision Skin" and are for plastic surgery and expensive.

Now that we know what we are looking for, let's learn how to properly rob a doctor's office!

PILFERING PILLS & PEN LIGHTS

There's a trick to everything, and several for looting. Here are a few to keep in mind:

While it's true that most doctors' offices will be ransacked after a catastrophe, don't be so quick to pass them by.   Unless on fire, they'll still have some goodies.

You'll find the medication sample closet and surgical supply cabinet stripped clean.   But remember when doctors go into a room to do minor procedures, we often stuff extra syringes, hypodermic needles, and packages of suture into our lab coats.   That way we won't have to leave the room and search for supplies we've forgotten.   But we rarely use them and often forget they are still in our coats. Only when sitting down at our desks, do we realize all this stuff is still in our pockets.   We will often throw these things into the back of one of our desk drawers.   Inevitably, some of these supplies will fall down beneath the drawers.   So take out the desk drawers, and search the floor.

You're likely to find loose packages of sample medications stuck between the drawers and their tracks; as well as needles, suture, and syringes scattered about on the floor.   But these little tidbits aren't why you're really here.

47

You are trying to find something you normally carry in your medical kit.   You're looking for a book!

Look around the office for small book called The Monthly Prescribing Reference.   It's a black booklet about the size of a TV guide.   Doctors get these free every month.   It has a concise summary of most common prescription medicines. It will tell you what a drug treats, what the typical dosage is, and of any common side effects.   If you cut your hand, it will tell you which antibiotic to take.

MPR

WHILE RUMMAGING THROUGH A MEDICAL OFFICE, GRAB COTTON BALLS, SWABS, GAZE, AND ESPECIALLY A MPR. COTTON BALLS ARE MORE VALUABLE AS TENDER FOR A FIRE, THAN FOR MEDICAL USES. AND THE MPR SUMMARIZES MEDICATIONS AND THEIR USES. IT'S LIKE GOLD!

Doctors are supposed to throw these away monthly when an updated version comes in the mail, but they rarely get around to it.   That means several are often floating around the office, sometimes even lodged under a supply cabinet or shimming the leg of an exam table.   Take the time to look, one is all you will need.

Ask your doctor for an old copy during your next checkup. They're usually happy give them away. While technically they go out of date every month, they're really good for five or ten years. This is because the new medications they're updated with, are not typically the kind you'll need in the field. Even if you're not putting together a medical kit, you may still want to get one for reference. Mothers want to know about the medicines prescribed for their children, and browsing through one will expand your medical knowledge. The publication is going digital, so you might also be able to download it from the internet.

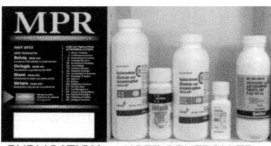 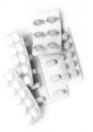

PUBLICATION IS GOING DIGITAL SOON   NOTE CONTROLLED "C" WITH II OR III INSIDE   EXAMPLES OF SAMPLES

Here's another trick: To keep up with regulations, doctors have to throw away outdated medical supplies. These include syringes, hypodermic needles, sample medications, and even gauze. They really hate to do this. They're expensive to replace, and many physicians feel the regulation is ridiculous. Most would much rather see them used in an emergency situation, than having to throw good supplies into the trash.

But unlike the case with The Monthly Prescribing Reference, some are unlikely to hand over supplies unless they know that they're bound for missionary work out of the country.   Then they're often eager to help.   Otherwise they feel there's just too much liability in giving them away, and they are right!   If they're willing, ask if they'd give you a call when updating their supplies.   Most are required by insurance companies, or the department of health, to update these.   Few physicians have ever been able to figure out how an Ace Bandage could go out of date.   But that's why there are government agencies... for the really important stuff!

Ask your physician if they would call you next time they are updating their supplies. They often have to throw out good supplies in order to comply with government regulations.

When I've given away sample medications or medical supplies for home medical kits, I'd give the patient a note written on a prescription pad.   It would read something like "these medications and supplies are for prescription use for this patient."   Then I'd put the person's name on top. This will usually keep you out of legal trouble if you get stopped.   Remember most police are likely to keep a home medical kit of their own, so many are understanding.

If you live in a very legally restrictive area or country, ask your doctor for a prescription to carry in your medical kit. It should say they are necessary for you to have, i.e. that they are prescriptions.

CONTROLLED SUBSTANCES

This classification is used by the DEA and includes narcotics, sedatives, and a few others. If a medication is controlled it will be marked with a capital "C" on the label with roman numerals inside.

C-II is the class most tightly controlled, and isn't available in sample form. C-III through C-V are less restricted, though doctors' offices are unlikely to keep them. This wasn't the case years ago. Back then most physicians kept pain medications on site. Now to keep them, clinics are required to have extra security and theft prevention measures. It's become an expensive hassle, as has repairing damage from break-ins. So most avoid it completely.

Doctors' offices are the least productive places to look for controlled substances!

Some preppers are dead set against firearms. I respect their stance on the issue, but encourage them to reconsider. There won't be anything else out there that can level the playing field. If nothing else, Less Than Lethal Weapons should be considered for personal and family protection. If you're going to use pepper spray, *then you must use the spray designed for bears* - not people (it's just not strong enough for live people _or_ zombies.)

The same is true of pharmaceutical representatives. They're the people that come into the doctor's office and squeeze in-between your physician and your appointment time. They used to give samples of pain medications and other controlled substances to doctors. But many of them were getting car jacked and beaten severely for the goodies people thought they had. Nowadays, if they're going to provide narcotic samples for doctors, they'll mail them directly from the company.

Side Note: Other Equipment to Look for or Buy Before the Big Day

Sometimes you may be able to find equipment in a doctor's office that will become invaluable later. In this side note discussion we'll be looking into a few inexpensive devices that can turn a zombie prepper into heavily valued commodity. We're going to learn to use them in detail as the chapters progress. For now know that with less than $150 investment you can fortify your medical kit sufficiently to diagnose, monitor, and treat most of the common and dangerous conditions the WWII preppers faced.

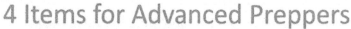

4 Items for Advanced Preppers

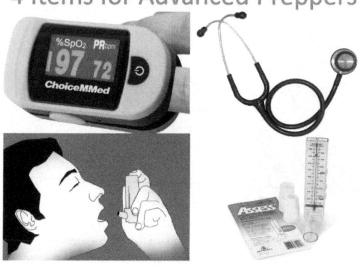

INFAMOUS DOCTORS & STETHOSCOPES

The first stethoscope was invented by a physician who wanted to live. As the story goes, he had been summoned to the queen's chamber for consultation. She'd been stricken ill with whatever respiratory bug was on special that century.

At this point in medical history, the common practice for listening to the heart and lungs involved the doctor placing his ear against the person's chest.   As you might imagine, being that close to the queen's knockers would have been incompatible with life.   The king would have gone medieval on the doctor!   A little quick thinking saved his skin.   He fashioned a hollow tube to bridge the gap.

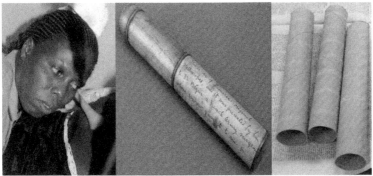

Shown center is the first stethoscope. Before the advent of this hollow wooden tube, the doctor had to put his ear to the sick persons chest. You can use a cardboard tube if you don't have a stethoscope. This also helps prevent you from catching the illness.

Modern stethoscopes can range from ten dollars, to over a thousand.   We recommend a $20 model.   With all of the equipment we will be discussing, it might be best to check eBay and others before heading over to Amazon.   At certain sites you can sometimes get more for less.

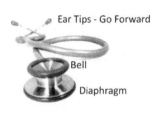

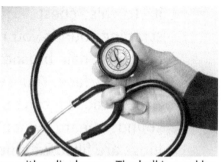

You'll only need a stethoscope with a diaphragm. The bell is used by cardiologists. We'll use the diaphragm for listening to lung sounds. Begin by inserting the ear tips into your ears with the tips pointing forward. Pivot the metal part around to switch from the bell to the diaphragm. Tap your finger on diaphragm to test. It should be loud.

The end of the stethoscope is divided into two parts: the bell, and the diaphragm. To switch from using one, to using the other, hold the tubing and rotate the metal portion. You'll hear a click when it snaps into place.

> **Tip**: If the person you're examining is outfitted with hair like Bigfoot, wet the diaphragm before putting it to his chest. This nulls the scraping sounds you might hear as his chest hair brushes against the plastic surface. You'll want to avoid this, because it can mimic the same sounds heard when a person's lungs are filled with fluid.

The bell picks up high-frequency sounds, like those produced by heart murmurs. We only need a stethoscope with a diaphragm. That's what's required for hearing the low-frequency noises associated with lung conditions.

After clicking the diaphragm into place, and putting the ear tips in your ears facing forward, tap on the plastic with your fingernail to make sure you're not still listening with the bell. You should hear a sharp loud pop when your fingernail strikes the diaphragm. If you do, you're good to go!

Pulse Oximeters & Blood of Color

Pulse oximeters were once very expensive. Now they're $20-60. The device shoots a beam of light into the person's bloodstream, then collects and analyzes the light reflected back. Comparing the color of blood in that gathered light, to an oxygen saturation chart, it estimates the amount of oxygen the person has in their bloodstream.

If a patient already has mild to moderate lung disease, emphysema for instance, a normal saturation (SpO2) will be above 90%. In healthy people it should be above 92%, and is generally in the range of 96-100% at rest.

Pulse Oximeter

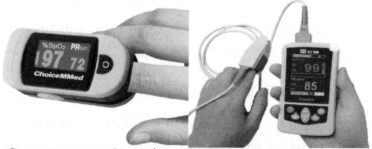

Once very expensive, pulse oximeters estimate the amount oxygen in the blood, & help you tell if the person is getting better or worse. They also tell you the persons heart rate.

Often referred to as a pulse ox, this instrument is useful to you in several ways. Increasing or decreasing oxygen saturation levels can help you determine if a person's condition is getting better or worse. It will also help you gauge if the quick acting treatments you'll be learning to provide are actually working, or if you should save your medicine for use elsewhere.

The person's heart rate (HR) is also displayed. 60-100 is normal, though it's faster the younger the child. The younger they are, the more rapid their pulse.

TIP: Tape extra batteries to the back of the Pulse Ox. You might be monitoring someone all night at times, which chews up batteries quickly!

In an adult, if the HR is above 100 bpm - a condition called tachycardia - the elevation generally reflects their body's attempt to improve oxygenation. We'll discuss this further in our pulmonary chapter.

PEAK EXPIRATORY FLOW METERS

First used to monitor and predict the severity of asthma attacks in children, peak flow meters can tell you a lot about a person's respiratory system.

Another $20 gizmo, these meters are labeled using either the English or Metric system, but typically not both. As much as I love to rail against the metric system, I've recently surrendered to its simplicity. The meter shown here uses the metric system.

We'll be discussing inhalers soon.   With the aid of a peak flow meter, you can determine if using an inhaler on a sick patient is going to be of benefit or not.

The Peak Expiratory Flow Meter

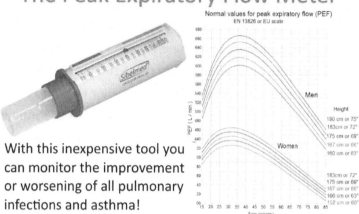

Normal values for peak expiratory flow (PEF)
EN 13826 or EU scale

With this inexpensive tool you can monitor the improvement or worsening of all pulmonary infections and asthma!

To use, start by removing and cleaning the transparent and disposable breathing tube the person wraps their lips around.   Then stick it back on.   Slide the red knob all the way back down to zero.   (Its current position in the photo is at 425, if you're having trouble finding it.)

Have the person take a big breath, then blow into the meter as quickly and with as much force possible.   The red slider will shoot upward and fix in place, registering the person's maximum expiratory flow.   Record that number and reference the height / age chart shown.   A graph like this will come with the product, showing values in English or Metric depending upon which you buy.

If a person already has asthma, chances are they'll know how it works. They might even have their own, along with an inhaler they're used to puffing on.

If a person has a lung infection, and they're having trouble breathing, measure their peak flow and record that number. Then have them take a dose of the inhaler we're going to recommend carrying in your kit. Wait a few minutes for it to take effect, then reset the meter and have them blow again. If they show improvement, you know they'll benefit from getting one or two puffs of the inhaler every 4 to six hours. If they don't, save your inhaler for later, it won't do anything helpful for that person.

Now let's look at more everyday equipment you'll want to scavenge or buy. These items are not specific to a pharmacy or doctor's office, but can often be found in diverse settings!

PICKING UP PICKUPS & FORCEPS

Pickups and forceps are essential for repairing wounds. The skin edges must be grasped somehow when sewing them back together. Cuts are common in the field, but you can fix them easily. And it's one of the most satisfying skills you can learn. It's something that should be taught in high school biology class - as should nutrition and basic pharmacology. Fears of liability will make sure that never happens.

Lacerations aren't as devastating as they first appear. A few bleed heavily, particularly in the face and scalp. Firm pressure held against the wound for a few minutes triggers blood vessels to clamp down, slowing the flow while initiating clotting mechanisms.

Cuts don't become infected as often as people think. Many times the worst consequence is a large and noticeable scar. Bleeding, risk of infection, and scar minimization are the reasons they need to be closed. When I say closed, I mean sutured back together.

> When suturing in the scalp, use antibiotic ointment, or even Vaseline, like you would hair gel. Comb the hair away from the cut. This helps prevent infection, and makes access to the wound easier.

Three things are needed: forceps, needle holders, and scissors.

Surgical forceps, often called pickups, look like large tweezers. They come in two basic styles: with and without teeth. Teeth are metal projections inside the jaws of forceps. They vary in size and are the type required for laceration repairs.

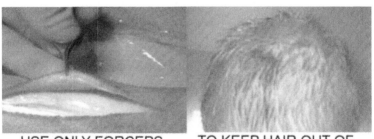

USE ONLY FORCEPS WITH TEETH TO PICK UP SKIN EDGES OR YOU WILL CRUSH THE TISSUE

TO KEEP HAIR OUT OF A SCALP WOUND WHILE SUTURING, COMB IT BACK WITH BACITRACIN

Forceps with teeth, also called pickups with teeth, are the only kind needed for your kit. The reason is purely mechanical. A tissue grasper with smooth or even textured jaws, must be squeezed together tightly, or it will lose hold on the skin edge. The excessive force will cause your fingers to fall asleep, and more important, destroy the tissue being held.

Extreme pressure causes something called "crush necrosis." Blood vessels in the area are crushed shut, causing the tissue to die. The reason it's problematic, is because bacteria thrive on dead tissue. The areas then become sources of infection. By using forceps with teeth, you can grab the tissue very gently, avoiding the whole problem.

This is why tweezers don't work for suturing. They're most useful for removing foreign objects, so be sure to include a set in your medical kit. If you're going to buy forceps, get those that are four or six inches long, they are the easiest to use.

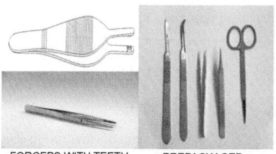

FORCEPS WITH TEETH
ABOVE - FORCEPS WITH
SERRATIONS BELOW

PREPACKAGED
SUTURE KIT WITH
FORCEPS

FORCEPS
WITHOUT TEETH
- AVOID THESE!

If you find yourself collecting instruments while moving from location to location, you can substitute forceps with other tools.

Sometimes needle nose pliers with deep serrations will work, just remember to be careful with the force you apply. Other times you can bend the flat ends of large tweezers inward, making teeth of your own. But the best way is to find strong stiff wire, and curl the end inward to make a hook. Then you can hook the skin edge you're working on, and pull it in the desired direction. I've made hooks like this in the past, and found them quite helpful.

Needle Nose Pliers & Wire

WHILE YOU'RE IN THE GARAGE, FIND NEEDLE NOSE PLIERS AND STIFF WIRE. SMALL WELDING RODS WORK WELL. BOTH CAN BE USED AS FORCEPS OR TISSUE HOOKS LATER.

Side Note: Suturing Shortcuts – Use a Straight Needle

If you choose to use a straight needle for closing skin gashes, then placing sutures is easy. This technique requires almost no equipment, and takes only minutes to learn and perform!

We discussed earlier how suturing needles come in many shapes and sizes, with most being curved into a half-circle. The type we'll be using for rapid closures are straight and flat at the end. They're convenient, because unlike with curved needles, you don't need any other instruments. And a thin package or two of suture on a straight needle takes up little room in your medical kit.

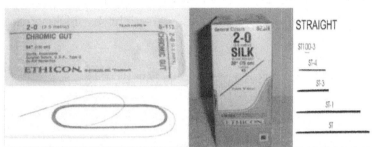

IF THERE ISN'T A PICTURE OF A NEEDLE SHOWN ON THE PACKAGE, IT CONTAINS SUTURE ONLY (TOP LEFT). STRAIGHT NEEDLE ON A 2-0 IS BEST TO HAVE

Pinch the skin edges together, run the straight needle through both side with a single pass, and pick up the suture ends. Tie them three or four times, cut off the excessive string, and move on to the next throw. Here's a video on the technique:

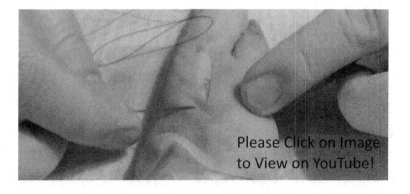

Please Click on Image to View on YouTube!

https://www.youtube.com/watch?v=VlsWyOM4rfI&feature=youtu.be

On our video channel you'll also find a video on how to close the wound quickly in one shot. Known as a "running suture," you save time by only cutting and tying only once, not every time a new throw is placed. This type of closure can also be make watertight by locking the running suture as you go!

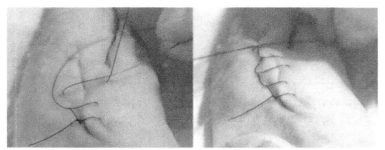

For a "water tight" running-locking suture, tie your first throw as usual. Now, take another bite and send the needle through, but don't pull it tight yet. Stop and run the needle though the loop you created from that second throw, then pull it tight. Repeat in 1cm intervals, and tie as usual at the end.

After watching our videos you'll be good to go. Additional straight needle suturing techniques can be found on The Prepper Pages YouTube channel.

There are some tools you'd like to have, and some tools you need to have. But arising above all others, is the grey roll of awesomeness gifted by the hand of God... Duct Tape! A favorite of zombie preppers everywhere:

TAPING LIFE BACK TOGETHER

You can use almost any tape to secure a dressing in place. But some cause skin damage when removed.

Don't wait until you see zombies in your backyard before putting a roll of duct tape in your BOB!

Surgical tape comes in a variety of styles, but the adhesive strength in each is different. If left on for long periods, duct tape will tear the skin when removed. Medical tapes are much gentler. Try to pilfer a few rolls of each for your bag. Otherwise you'll end up buying an entire box of each. After examining the strength of each type, choosing the right kind for the wound you're treating will come naturally.

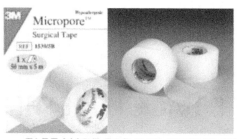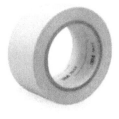

TAPE MADE FOR USE ON THE SKIN COMES IN
PAPER, RUBBERY, AND CLOTH TYPES - NEVER RUN
ANY OF THESE CIRCUMFERENTIALLY AROUND A LIMB,
YOU MAY CAUSE EXCESSIVE SWELLING THAT WAY

While Running from Zombies...

IF YOU CUT YOURSELF WHILE RUNNING FROM THE HORDES, QUICKLY TAPE THE CUT SHUT AND SUTURE IT LATER. DO THE SAME TO MAKE A SPLINT IF YOU HAVE A SPRAIN OR BREAK AND NEED TO KEEP MOVING.

*When fixing a bandage into position, **never wrap a single piece of tape all the way around a limb like you would with an elastic bandage.*** Tape doesn't stretch like they do. Consequently, it acts like a tourniquet and cuts off the blood supply. If you need to wrap tape completely around a limb, tear it into strips first. Then apply it like you would to a plastic sheet covering a window you're painting around.

There are special circumstances exempt from this rule. Taping a sprained ankle for stability is one example. We'll discuss others shortly.

If you don't have skin or surgical tape, and are rummaging for anything you available, don't bother with electrical or masking tape. They will fall off just as soon as the person starts to sweat.

Sometimes you'll find yourself falling back to duct tape to keep dressings attached for extended periods. Normally you'll remove it once you're safe and starting definitive treatment. But if forced to use it for longer spans, tear the duct tape into small pieces and secure the dressing as usual. But the next time you change the bandage, put the new pieces of tape on areas of skin that have not previously been used. By rotating where the tape is placed, you limit the amount of skin damage it creates.

Duct tape prevents blindness!

SNOW BLINDNESS

Duct tape has endless uses, one of which is the prevention of a particular type of blindness...snow blindness. It's like a sunburn of the eye. Usually not noticed until several hours afterword, it occurs from exposure to sunlight

Tip: A pair of sunglasses should be included in every bug-out bag.

that's been reflected off ice, snow, or less commonly sand and sea.   Fresh snow reflects about 80% of the sun's ultraviolet (UV) radiation.   Sea foam and beach sand reflect less.   Snow blindness is particularly problematic at high altitudes and in Polar Regions.

Symptoms include increased tears and scratchy pain; it feels like having sand in your eyes.   Pain and tears will make you functionally blind and unable to navigate over land.

It can be prevented two ways: By wearing eye protection that blocks ultraviolet radiation.   Or by wearing slit goggles.

Sunglasses with UV filters are not always available. Lacking this modern convenience, Inuit peoples were able to solve the problem by carving goggles with a thin horizontal slit.   You can emulate this design by making a similar pair out of duct tape.

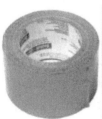
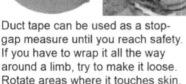
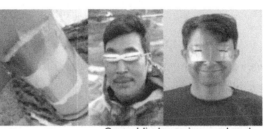

Duct tape can be used as a stop-gap measure until you reach safety. If you have to wrap it all the way around a limb, try to make it loose. Rotate areas where it touches skin.

Snow blindness is a real and dangerous problem if you don't have sunglasses. Use duct tape to make a pair with thin slits like the Inuit have.

If a person has snow blindness, remove them from sunlight and cover their eyes with patches. Administer pain relief while the patient rests. Cool wet compresses can help, but dropping lidocaine or another anesthetic into them inhibits healing. The pain and blurriness typically resolves in 24–72 hours. Further injury can be avoided by making duct tape glasses and wearing them whenever in high exposure environments.

Duct tape for snow glasses? Did you see that one coming? We wouldn't have. Now let's see what else we can MacGyver on the fly!

SLINGING BACK SPLINTS & SWATHS

A sling is a dressing that ties around a person's neck and supports their injured arm. It allows the extremity to rest in front of their body as it heals. A swath is something that affixes the sling to the person's trunk, thereby preventing further injuries.

Splints are different. They can be thought of as makeshift casts that try to prevent motion in broken bones or sprained joints. Learning to improvise a sling, swath, and splint is easy.

All three are necessary for a complete kit. But you can save space in your supply bag by learning to tie a sling from a towel or specialized bandage. There are a few short YouTube videos that show you how to do this. Better, you can buy something called a "triangular bandage," a device that can also be used as a pressure dressing.

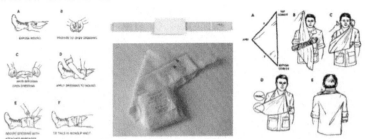

Pressure dressings can come prepackaged, and are sometimes sold as surplus military supplies. They can be made with 4x4s and tightly wrapped elastic, or inelastic and triangular bandages.

Inexpensive and capable of treating multiple conditions, they take up little room. They come with a safety pin in the package, and can be folded to the size you need for quick and effective arm immobilization.

Triangular bandages are typically made from muslin, but many other non-stretch materials can be used. Pants, ponchos, fatigues, blankets and towels all work well. Tear, cut or fold the material into a triangular shape to get started. Find something around you now that might work and follow the folding patterns shown in the diagram. After you do it once, you'll remember it.

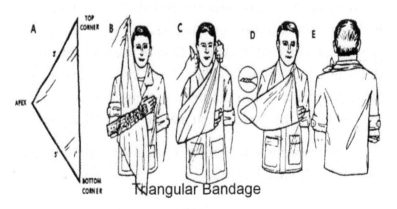

Triangular Bandage

Instructions for Constructing a Triangular Bandage

A. First, insert the material under the injured arm so that the arm is in the center, the apex of the material is beyond the elbow, and the top corner of the material is over the shoulder of the injured side.

B. Carefully position the forearm so the hand is slightly higher than the elbow by about 10 degrees

C. Next, bring the lower portion of the material over the injured arms so the bottom corner goes of the shoulder of the uninured side.

D. Bring the top corner behind the patient's neck.

E. Tie the two corners together so that your knot doesn't slip. The knot should fit into the empty space at the side of the neck resting on the patient's good side.

Splints can be fashioned with a flat wood board you've foraged, or with thick cardboard folded in layers. If you're putting together your supplies, a few companies sell versatile and malleable splits. They're usually made from a metal like aluminum, and are lined on the inside with cushioning foam. You can bend the metal into the shape you need, and then secure it in place with an elastic wrap.

Lightweight splints come in all sizes, including some made for individual fingers.

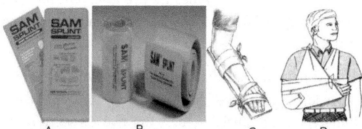

A   B   C   D

Pre-manufactured splints are easy to use (A and B). They can be made from folded newspapers, magazines, or light flat boards (C). Note that two triangular bandages were used here, the first as a sling, and the second as a swath (D).

FINDING NEEDLES & SYRINGES IN A HAYSTACK

These days needles and syringes seem easier to find than street drugs. Sometimes they're given out for free, though it might require standing in a community clinic line for a few hours.

Syringes are classified by the number of CC's or ml's they hold. But the abbreviation "CC," for cubic centimeters, is no longer used. The two C's were being confused with two zeros, leading to accidental overdoses. So medicine switched units to milliliters (ml's.) This conversion is easily made, because 1 CC is equal to 1 ml.

You need two sizes of syringes, one for injections, and one for wound irrigation. Three to five milliliter syringes work best for injections, and 10-20 ml work best for washing out wounds.

The most important thing about cleaning a contaminated wound is the water pressure used while washing it out. In the emergency room we try to use a force equivalent to at least 10 pounds per square inch. The process begins by filling up a 10 ml syringe with saline, and attaching an 18 gauge catheter to its end. The physician squirts it into the wound quickly, refills the syringe, and repeats the process until a minimum of 250 ml's have been used.

In the field, just fill the syringe with saline or tap water, and shoot it into the wound as rapidly as possible. Repeat this several times.   Tap water has been shown to be as effective as sterile saline, particularly if you mix in an antiseptic.   We'll talk more about wounds and irrigation later.   For now let's discuss the uses of smaller syringes.

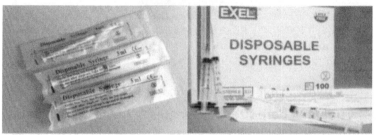

Disposable syringes come in 1ml, 2ml, 5ml, 10ml, and larger. It's easiest to buy the ones that come with a needle, usually a 21g (gauge) needle 1.25" long. A box of 25, 5ml x 21g x 1.25 syringes costs about $10. Some syringes are marked ml/cc.

Syringes come in two main varieties: those with, and those without needles in the package.   Most small syringes, like those designed for injecting insulin, come with a very small non-removable needle.   Two milliliter and five milliliter syringes can come with detachable needles if you order them that way.   Insulin syringes can be very helpful when injecting local anesthetic around wounds, but only when a small amount is needed.   They're more comfortable because their small needle size decreases the patient's pain during the injection.   The drawback is that they can only hold 1ml of medicine at a time.

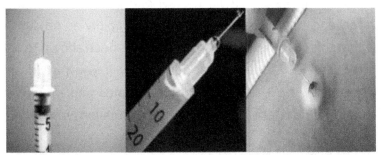

Insulin syringes only hold 1ml of fluid, and the needle is not removable. They are marked 10, 20, 30, ect. that denote 0.1, 0.2, 0.3 mililiters respectively. They are good for tick removal.

Hypodermic needles come in a bewildering assortment of bore sizes and lengths. In the United States, their size is based on the gauge system. The larger the number, the smaller the bore. A 30 gauge needle is the smallest and the size that comes attached to insulin syringes. They can be used for special applications like tick removal, which we'll discuss in depth a little later.

When a 3ml, 5ml, or 10ml syringe comes with a needle, it's typically a 21 gauge. This is a good size for drawing up medications from multi-dose vials. If you want less pain during the injection, you can buy 25 or 27 gauge needles, and swap them out for the 21 gauge that comes in the package.

When you buy supplies: syringes, needles, tape, suture or whatever, they often come in boxes of 20, 50 or 100. It's sometimes best to make a list of everything you need, then go in with a group of people on the purchase. Divvying these bulk supplies up amongst your group can save a lot of money and benefit everyone.

Hypodermic needles also come in different lengths. ¾ inch is a useful for injecting anesthetics. You shouldn't have any trouble finding them for sell on the Internet. The drawback is you'll often have to buy an entire box.

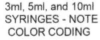
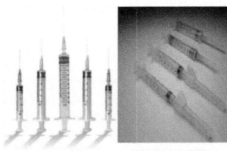
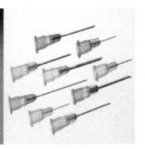

| 3ml, 5ml, and 10ml SYRINGES - NOTE COLOR CODING | SYRINGES WITH SINGLE USE NEEDLES | VARIOUS NEEDLE LENGTHS AND GAUGES |

If you're having difficulty buying needles and syringes, it might be easiest to talk to your physician. If you tell them that you're using these items for an emergency medical kit, many won't have a problem writing a prescription for the supplies you'll need. This goes for medicines as well. Despite a general reputation for poor bedside manner, most physicians are caring individuals and want to help you out if they can. Remember they're likely have their own emergency medical kits, so many already know what you're going to need.

Don't be afraid to ask!

INTRAVENOUS NEEDLES & CATHETERS FOR THE HOME AND OFFICE

Did you know that the intravenous catheter (I.V.) has been credited with saving more people than antibiotics? This factoid surprises people.   Most think that penicillin and sulfa are what turned the tide in humanities war against germs.   But in reality the I.V. saved the most people.   Back then most died from dehydration before their infection had the chance to kill them.   This is still occurring in countries stricken with Ebola, and explains why the mortality rate there is so high.   Most don't have access to I.V.'s.   So learning to put one is time well spent.

Many have learned to do this from watching YouTube videos; including a scripted character on AMC's Breaking Bad.   But if it seems impractical or overwhelming, you might be able to find a nurse or paramedic to teach you. Another alternative is to host a talk or seminar by someone willing to teach a group of like-mined individuals.

Bags of I.V. fluid usually cost doctors about a dollar each.   The problem with a liter of normal saline is that it takes up a lot of room in your medical kit.   And several bags can get heavy. There are other draw backs. You must know what fluids to give, and they must remain sterile.

Administering the wrong fluid could kill the person. Finally, the I.V. bags expire quickly, and this is one of the few times where the expiration date is critically important.

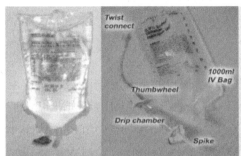

SPECIFICATION

FOR AN I.V. YOU NEED BAGS OF NORMAL SALINE, CONNECTION TUBING AND I.V. CATHETERS

CATHETERS COME IN MANY SIZES AND ARE COLOR CODED

If you're going to learn medical skills for the field, we recommend suturing, I.V. insertion, and CPR in that order. For zombie preppers, it might be even more important to learn how to administer intravenous fluids than to learn CPR.

By the time people need CPR, unless it's because they are choking, they're usually not going to survive anyway. In a normal non-apocalyptic situation, CPR can be extremely useful. In these instances the ill person can be transported to a hospital for definitive treatment. But care like that probably won't be available in the environment we're discussing. Hospitals are likely to reorganize into something like aid stations located in old houses, much like they were on the American Frontier.

82

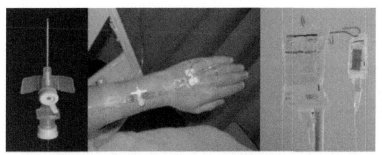

Intravenous catheter insertion is a skill the prepper should learn. WikiHow and YouTube both provide instructional videos and materials.

Even if you don't learn how to put in I.V's, the plastic catheters covering the needles have many potential uses. If you get a large one, 14, 16, or 18 gauge, you can save the plastic catheter sheaths and throw away the needles.

Bags of I.V. fluid can be warmed and used as hot water bottles, or something soft to rest an injured extremity on. They can also be taped in place and used as a comfortable pressure dressing.

This outer sheath can then be hooked up to a syringe. You can use this set up to irrigate wounds, or flush out ears occluded by wax. For both, it's far superior to using a syringe alone.   It increases the pressure of the fluid coming out, and directs the stream more effectively.

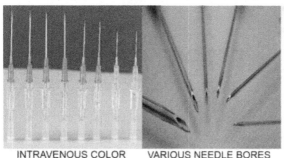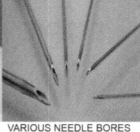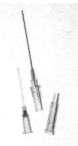

| INTRAVENOUS COLOR CODED CATHETERS - NOTE IT'S A PLASTIC "TUBE" OVER VARIOUS SIZED NEEDLES | VARIOUS NEEDLE BORES WITH THE OVERLYING PLASTIC CATHETERS REMOVED | ANGIOCATHETER WITH THE FLEXIBLE OUTER PLASTIC "TUBE" REMOVED |

If you're going to buy bags of IV fluid, buy normal saline.   They're marked "NS 0.9%," and have a few other uses.   You can use it as sterile irrigation for wounds, or heat the bags and use them as warm packs for sprains and strains.

Side Note: Other Essential I.V. Catheter Modifications

Later in this book we'll be discussing how to tweak I.V.'s for treating a life-threatening condition called pneumothorax.

In that disease, the space between the lung and chest wall fills with air causing the lung to collapse.   Commonly resulting from rib fractures, pneumothorax is almost always present after a bullet or other object pierces a person's chest.   It's something of a trick to treat.   We're going to

84

discuss the particulars later, but for now we'll show you what you'll need for a fast and easy fix.

In the hospital setting, the preferred treatment for evacuating the trapped air involves placing something called a chest tube.   A procedure few primary care physicians feel comfortable performing, and one taking surgical residents a year or two to master.   We'll be using the much easier technique of needle decompression.   For performing it you'll need the following:

Making a Decompression Needle

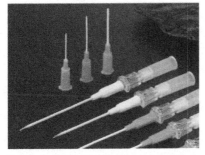 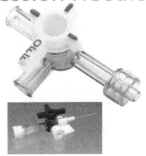

To make a thoracostomy needle for decompressing a pneumo-thorax, find the largest bore I.V. catheter you can. Insert it into the anterior chest wall between the 2nd & 3rd ribs, halfway between the nipple and sternum. Pull the needle out so only the plastic remains. Attach a closed stopcock or syringe. Open the valve every 15 minutes or so to release the air.

Have you seen the Clooney movie *Three Kings*?   As I recall, Marky Mark takes one to the chest and Clooney saves the day by sticking one of these in him.   Perhaps it's not the best training video, but it illustrates the basic idea.

We'll link to some real instructional videos later in an upcoming chapter. For now, you'll want to find the largest bore I.V. catheter - 14 gauge if possible – and a closeable valve called a stopcock. If you don't have this valve, either attach a syringe or improvise a one-way valve. Again, more later!

Now that we have that out of the way, let's move on to something fun... looting!

THE SCIENCE OF LOOTING

Rule 18- *"It's better to seek forgiveness than ask permission"* - Leroy Jethro Gibbs, NCIS

This is a good time to talk about the leftovers in a drugstore after it's been looted. Often people leave important items, not realizing their value. Other times the store will have been stripped clean, and not worth entering. You want to get into these places after the angry mobs are finished, but before they're set on fire. This timing is the art of looting, though at this stage it's more like hurried rummaging. Think carefully about what you'll be looking for before entering the store. These aren't places you want to be in for a second longer than necessary.

You may be able to find bags of intravenous fluid, particularly if the pharmacy is near a hospital. Those nearby often mix and compound medicines for hospitals and doctors' offices. Stores like Rite Aid don't, but are more accessible. They aren't crowded by hospital traffic. But pharmacies are a low yield venture in the first place. You'll want to rifle through a pet store to find the good stuff. We'll talk more about that later!

You might think the most important things to find while searching a pharmacy are pain pills and antibiotics. Many people think this way, and it can work to your advantage. While antibiotics can sometimes make the difference between living and dying, narcotics seem to be even more valued. Looters are usually focused on these, overlooking items of real value.

> *Be aware that if people know that you have Vicodin or other pain pills, many won't think twice before shooting you and snatching them.*

Important things you can recover from a looted pharmacy include: multivitamins, electrolyte mixes, cotton balls, Betadine, and Vaseline. Any global disaster is likely to last a long time, and malnutrition becomes a real problem. Good health requires both calories and vitamins. Because people don't think this way, they will loot narcotics first, antibiotics second, batteries and expensive looking items third. Often the multivitamins and electrolyte mixes aren't touched.

<u>Side Note</u>: Mineral Deficiencies - Iron

No doubt about it... *children can be gross.* One of my favorite behaviors of these little rascals is called is Pica. The tendency of children to eat dirt. There's a variant of Pica where the child chews ice instead, and to me that's a little less disturbing.

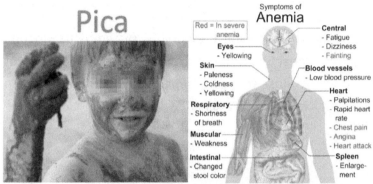

When children eat dirt, or sometimes ice, it can be a neurological response to low levels of Iron or Zinc in their blood. This might indicate they have an underlying anemia.

The dirt eating version was a common in the children of WWII, suggesting many may have been anemic. Pica is thought to be an adaptive evolutionary response developed millennia ago. The behavior seems to reactivate in anemic children, and tells them they need to acquire iron by eating dirt. It appears we still have some worm genes and behavior in us.

You probably won't have the ability to check for anemia in these children. So if yours are eating dirt, it's best to assume they're anemic and to start treating them with iron and zinc supplements. The behavior will eventually stop, hopefully before they ingest some ugly parasite living in the soil they find yummiest.

Side Note: Mineral Deficiencies - Salt

Salt is essential if the nervous system is to function properly. Reaction times and mental clarity suffer without it. If you're close to a coast line, it can be harvested from the sea if a mine is not available.

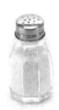 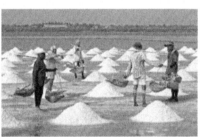

Critically missing from many prepper lists is salt. Every cell depends upon having a steady supply. Nerves cannot fire, and your brain cannot work, without common table salt. So important to life, it was often traded ounce for ounce with gold in the ancient world. Don't forget about this in your preps!

In antiquity the names of towns where salt could be found ended with the suffix –wich or Hall. Greenwich being a well-known example. During a prolonged disaster in the United States we'll be hard pressed to find a natural or adequate supply, so it's best to have a hefty amount already stashed. After a thirty year war on sodium in

America, coupled with the large quantities found in our everyday food, it's an absolute necessity that's often overlooked and rarely considered in many prepper lists.

Side Note: Ricketts & Livers

Not known for an abundance of sunbathing beaches, the English coastline can be a gray and dreary manufacturer of depression. *Even when it's not raining explosives.*

Sunlight is essential to the health of a child. Without it the well-known reaction between sun and skin doesn't occur. And the vitamin D necessary for strong and straight bones cannot be made in sufficient amounts.

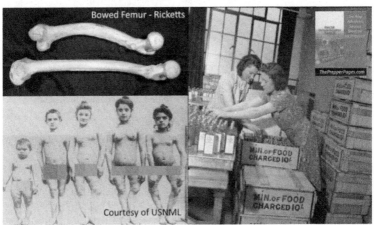

Children living in northern latitudes need as much sunlight as possible to synthesize vitamin D through their skin, otherwise their bones soften & bow (Ricketts). In WWII, shelters equaled deficiency, & so the Food Ministry had to rely on cod liver oil.

With the aid of the pasty white skin many of us Caucasians sport, we're usually able to eke out enough to make a living - and life goes on.

But that uncertain line was crossed in WWII when people were forced to live in subterranean bomb shelters. In those instances you can bank on Ricketts sweeping through and stealing the strength and structural integrity of a child's rapidly growing bones. The only available solution back then was to extract vitamin D from something that produced a lot of it, then give it to children orally. And so the Cod, or rather its liver, was drafted into service by the British Empire.

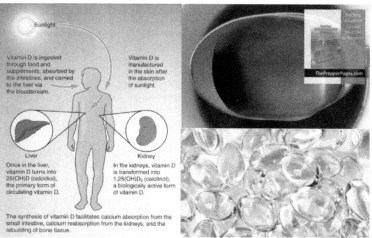

In lue of adequate sunlight, a tablespoon of Cod liver oil was given to every British school-age child a day. We're told it was a tough sell. So it's better to give it to our children in pill form.

For zombie preppers, finding Vitamin D capsules in a looted pharmacy or stocking them at your BOL is easier.

FINAL ITEMS TO SEARCH FOR IN PHARMACIES

Before you leave, look around to see if any antiseptics are left. Over the counter solutions fall into three groups: alcohol, hydrogen peroxide, and Betadine.

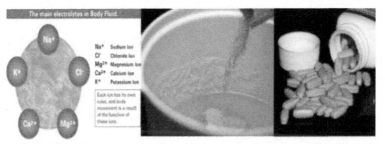

Good health and wound healing require calories, vitamins, and electrolytes. Powdered electrolytes take up little room. Multivitamins for children should be included in your kit.

Isopropyl alcohol, also called rubbing alcohol, is the most plentiful. This form of alcohol cannot be ingested without the risk of severe bodily harm. Ethanol is the type of alcohol you can both drink and use to cleanse wounds. As a general rule, if you can light it on fire, it's strong enough to use as an antiseptic. Weaker than that, and it may not be as effective.

There are a couple of disadvantages to using rubbing alcohol. First, it hurts like hell when poured into an open wound. Second, it's not an agent that kills bacteria; we say that it's not "bactericidal." In a way that's helpful. Because if it doesn't kill bacterial cells, then it also means that it won't kill the person's healthy cells lining the wound. You want to keep these alive, so they can replicate and fill-in the injury.

Betadine is the most important antiseptic, because it can also be used to sterilize water for drinking. A little in concentrated form goes a long way.

Alcohol may not destroy viruses, unless it's very concentrated. But this isn't important for most skin lacerations, because viruses don't usually cause wound infections.

BETADINE

The nuclear weapon of over-the-counter antiseptics. Betadine contains Iodine and has multiple uses. A small concentrated bottle takes up less room than rubbing alcohol, but kills indiscriminately. If you pour it into a wound, it will destroy both the germs - and your healthy tissue. This can be reduced by diluting the solution with saline or sterile water.

Bacteria thrive in injured cells. The dead material offers a rich energy source and media for them to replicate in. As a helpful rule, use dilute Betadine if you're treating a fresh wound, and full strength in a wound that's infected.

If you're using it to sterilize the skin before doing a procedure, you must let it dry first. Betadine's effectiveness is doubled only after it has dried! If you're preparing the skin before cutting out something lodged in it, or cleaning the edges before suturing them closed, don't begin cutting until the solution has dried.

HYDROGEN PEROXIDE

The last antiseptic we'll be discussing is hydrogen peroxide. It can be poured into a wound at low concentrations (3-5%) and has the advantage of not stinging. It can also be used to disinfect water, but this requires higher concentrations. It's bactericidal and easy to find. More uses of Betadine and hydrogen peroxide will be discussed in the chapter on water purification.

Droppers

MOVE THROUGH A DRUG-STORE QUICKLY, IT'S A DANGEROUS PLACE TO BE. FIRST LOOK FOR ANY BOTTLE THAT HAS A DROPPER, YOU'LL NEED THE DROPPER TO STERILIZE WATER LATER. THEN LOOK FOR BETADINE, VITAMINS, AND ELECTROLYTES. ANY ANTISEPTICS OR IV FLUIDS ARE A BONUS. LEAVE QUICKLY!

In the early stages, it can be difficult to tell if a wound is infected. If it's markedly red, warm, tender, draining non-clear fluid, or if the person has a fever with no other obvious cause, then treat it as if it's infected.

The last three medicines to look for on the grocery or Wal-Mart floor, are Ibuprofen, Tylenol and Primatene Mist Inhalers.

Ibuprofen may be better than Tylenol if you have to choose. This is because Tylenol is not an anti-inflammatory. It can treat mild to moderate pain and relieve fever. But if you take it for a sprained ankle or similar injury, it won't treat the underlying inflammation.

ALBUTEROL & PRIMATENE MIST INHALERS – PUFFING & HUFFING AEROSOLIZED ADRENALIN

Having an inhaler in your kit can make all the difference in treating allergic reactions, asthma, and a number of other lung infections and conditions. Albuterol being the one you'd really want. But it's available by prescription only, unless you get it through the internet or by other creative means.

If you cannot find albuterol, you can get the over-the-counter (OTC) form called Primatene Mist.   Like Albuterol, also known as Proventil, Primatene Mist is a bronchodilator. It relaxes the muscles surrounding the airways.   Opening them to different degrees depending upon the illness a person has.   Its major drawback lies in its harsh side effect profile.   It can raise a person's heart rate and cause palpitations, or "fluttering of the heart."   It also tends to make the person shaky and nervous.   It's basically inhaled adrenalin!

Albuterol is much safer and has fewer side effects. For many of us, it remains something of a mystery why it's still by prescription only, and why Primatene mist isn't.

Just about any condition that causes wheezing will improve with either of these inhalers.   By no means are they the only puffers out there.   However, the others are usually either aerosolized steroids or medications designed to prevent asthma attacks.   So they're not of much use to you when you're trying to treat someone with an acute illnesses.

Inhalers

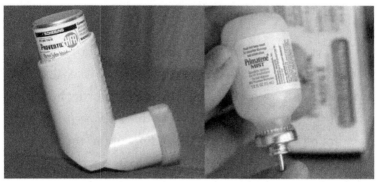

Wheezing most often occurs with asthma, but can also be present with allergic reations and infections like bronchitis. Albuterol is Rx. Primatene is OTC, but has more side effects.

We've saved the most important point about inhalers for last.   And that is that hardly anyone uses one correctly. (In the appendix we've placed an illustration with directions on how to properly use one.)   This means more often than not, the medication sprays the back of a person's throat and never makes it into their lungs where it's needed.   Luckily, "there's an app for that."

SPACERS & AEROCHAMBERS – LIFE SAVERS FOR THE UNCOORDINATED

In the 1990s the improper use of inhalers meant many children, some with life-threatening asthma, were being undertreated.   In response a device called a spacer, or sometimes an AeroChamber, was marketed for use with most types of inhaled medications.

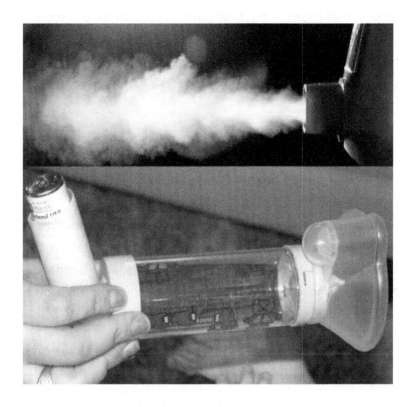

This meant trying to time your inhalation just perfectly so a mist, like the one shown on top, could make its way into the deepest recesses of your lungs was no longer a problem. One spray of the inhaler is delivered into the chamber at a time. The person begins by hooking the inhaler into the spacer, sprays a burst, then puts their mouth to the other end and starts breathing deeply. After a minute or two the procedure is repeated with a 2nd puff - *if necessary.*

Hauling around a full-sized spacer in your kit can take up precious room. But that's not a problem for a prepper! If room is an issue, either buy a collapsible model, or study the design and plan to make one of your own from scavenged parts when you need it.

MORE ON EXPIRATION DATES

You can go hog wild acquiring all sorts of medicines for your med bag, but most will expire without having been used. This might not be anything more than a theoretical problem for most pills and supplies. Many question the validity of expiration dates on medicines and bandages. Neither of these are equivalent to the expiration date on a gallon of milk, or a vial of insulin.

Tylenol can relieve pain and fever, but is not an anti-inflammatory medication.

While the date on some medications is essential, the idea of a strict date being extended to all is unreasonable. Many of us feel it's used as a last chance by companies to force people into endlessly buying their product. If your ibuprofen is 10 years old, then in an emergency you might need to take one and a quarter instead of one. For most medications, particularly those that are over-the-counter, the expiration date probably doesn't count for much... not after zombies are running around everywhere.

Let's talk about more cool toys next!

SPECIAL SUPPLIES FOR COMMON INJURIES & INFECTIONS

QUICKCLOT

There are a few specialized items you may want for your kit. One great product is Quickclot 25. It's used to control bleeding and runs about $10.00 a package. You simply empty its contents into a bleeding wound, and apply a pressure dressing. It won't work for complex wounds, like those involving organs. But in the extremities it's an easy way to stop hemorrhaging. It also has antibiotic properties, killing two birds with one stone. You have to be careful with some of these products. Many are applied in the field for combat injuries, but then have to be irrigated out when the patient arrives in the operating room. So read the product description or watch a YouTube video on their use before buying.

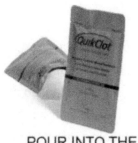

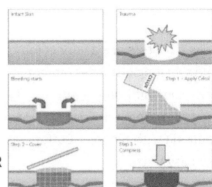

**POUR INTO THE
WOUND THEN COVER
WITH A DRESSING**

MOLE FOAM, 2ND SKIN, AND DUCT TAPE

Two other well-designed products are mole foam and 2nd skin. These padded adhesive materials protect blisters from further rubbing. Similar products are available in generic form. All are especially useful, because blisters from prolonged walking are among the most common injuries you'll encounter.

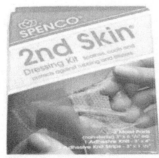

GREAT FOR TREATING BLISTERS,
A COMMON INJURY IN THE FIELD

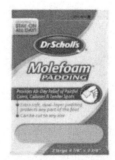

DrScholl's MOLEFOAM
ALSO WORKS WELL

Blisters are a very common when people are forced to travel long distances on foot. They can occur anywhere, and from different injuries. Typically they're caused by forceful rubbing or friction. Most fill with clear fluid, but some fill with blood. Both types can become infected but are easy to treat.

When they occur on locations other than the feet, the recommendation is to leave them intact until they burst on their own. The overlying skin protects the underlying tissue from becoming infected. But on the foot this recommendation becomes impractical. Here you'll want to take a sterile needle and puncture the blister in a direction parallel to the skin. Make the hole as small as possible, but evacuate the fluid. After draining, place triple antibiotic ointment on the area, then cover it with a dressing.

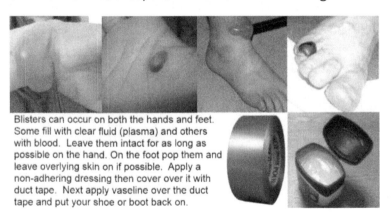

Blisters can occur on both the hands and feet. Some fill with clear fluid (plasma) and others with blood. Leave them intact for as long as possible on the hand. On the foot pop them and leave overlying skin on if possible. Apply a non-adhering dressing then cover over it with duct tape. Next apply vaseline over the duct tape and put your shoe or boot back on.

> *You can use the Duct tape*
> *Vaseline trick for anywhere*
> *rubbing and chafing is a*
> *problem. Backpack straps*
> *and web belts are common*
> *culprits.*

Since the blister formed from abnormal friction, you will want to reduce the rubbing as best possible. Place a non-adhering dressing over the area and cover it with duct tape. Usually duct tape is much too hard on the skin, but on the foot the skin is thicker and can handle the adhesive. Duct tape can be made into a nearly frictionless surface with petroleum jelly. Simply cover the outer layer of the duct tape with Vaseline or ointment, and put your shoe or boot back on. This should remedy the situation until you get to your destination and have time to heal.

PREPACKAGED PRESSURE DRESSINGS

Israeli Bandages are prepackaged field expedient dressings. Also called "The Emergency Bandage," they're designed for stopping bleeding from traumatic injuries in emergency situations. They were used first during the NATO peacekeeping operations in Bosnia and Herzegovina. Invented by an Israeli military medic, they were nicknamed "Israeli bandages" by soldiers and have become the dressing of choice for the U.S. Army.

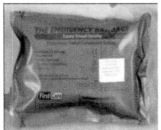

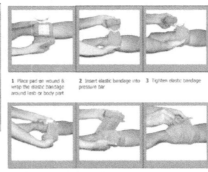

1 Place pad on wound & wrap the elastic bandage around limb or body part

2 Insert elastic bandage into pressure bar

3 Tighten elastic bandage

4 Pull back – forcing pressure bar down onto pad

5 Wrap elastic bandage tightly over pressure bar and wrap over all edges of pad

6 Secure hooking ends of closure bar into elastic bandage

Israeli Bandage

They're inexpensive at six dollars each, and come with application instructions like those shown above. The instructions are in English, but the best way to learn to apply them may be by watching YouTube videos.

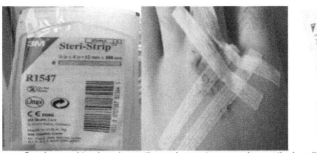

Can be used to close lacerations when sutures are impractical or difficult. Steri-Strips come in a variety of widths. They are designed to be used with an adhesive like that shown in the upper right corner. Betadine will work also. Remember to let both dry before applying the strips.

STERI-STRIPS

The last of the must have items are "Steri-Strips." They look like little pieces of tape adherent to a square of wax paper. Used to close wounds that might not require sutures, they stick to the skin and approximate the margins.

Often physicians will place steri-strips over the sutures they've put in to reinforce the repair. They come with an adhesive that you're supposed to apply to the skin first, but often applying Betadine will work just as well. You can close a laceration very quickly this way. And as with most other items, they never actually go out of date.

Eat a light lunch, next up is every manner of grossness!

WOUNDING ABSCESSES

Any kind of mishap can unfold in the field. Most common are sprains, strains, and wounds that either need to be closed, or that have become infected.

> *Abscesses must be drained if*
> *they are to heal. Antibiotics*
> *alone won't work.*

It takes a couple of days after an injury for an infection to develop. When limited to the skin and some of the fat below, an infection looks and feels like an excessively tender inflamed area. One that may be tense and draining foul smelling fluid. But when you feel around the area, there shouldn't be anything underneath this reddened wound. If you feel a ball like mass, it indicates that a fluid collection or abscess has developed.

Sometimes there isn't a recognizable break in the skin over an abscess, but the skin will be red and you'll be able to feel a tender mass that shouldn't be there. If there isn't any redness or tenderness, and the mass has developed slowly over time, then it probably isn't an abscess, it's likely a lipoma.

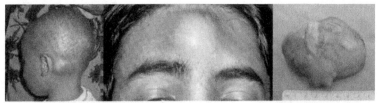

A lipoma can look like an abscess, but there's no redness, and minimal to no tenderness.

Lipomas are non-cancerous fatty growths.

Abscesses must be drained to heal.   You have to cut them open with a scalpel, a procedure called drainage.   Of course you'll want to numb the overlying skin first.   The particulars of injectable anesthetics are covered in the next chapter.

Many people think that strong antibiotics alone will cure an abscess.   But this rarely happens.   Antibiotics can't completely treat abscesses, because it's hard for them to enter the infected cavity.

In order to work, they have to be delivered through blood stream, and abscesses don't have a blood supply running through them.   They may prevent an infection from spreading, but alone they won't cure the problem.

I know this whole subject is about as sick as it gets. We would have left it out if abscesses weren't so common. Just remember to treat this condition, you'll have to open up the collection by cutting over the top with a sharp blade. Just one incision won't do.   You'll want to make two, forming a cut that resembles a crus or "X."

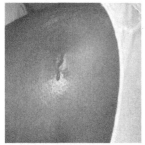
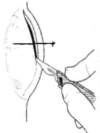
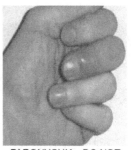

ABSCESSES MAY DRAIN SPONTANEOUSLY, BUT STILL MUST BE OPENED

DON'T STOP WITH A SIMPLE INCISION, MAKE A SECOND PERPENDICULAR

PARONYCHIA. DO NOT INCISE THE SKIN. SLIDE THE BLADE IN-BETWEEN THE NAIL AND SKIN.

Studies have repeatedly shown that leaving a drain in an abscess cavity is as effective as giving antibiotics for resolving the infection.

Even well trained physicians make the mistake of using a single slit. But then the skin will seal over too quickly, and the infected fluid will re-accumulate. When you make a cruciate incision, it'll take two or three days before spontaneously closing, thereby providing time for it to drain completely. Best of all, releasing the built up pressure will give immediate pain relief.

After you're done, mix saline and Betadine into a basin, and draw the solution up into a large syringe. Use it to irrigate out the cavity. For large abscesses it's best to leave in some sort of drain in, or to lightly pack the defect with gauze. An easy way to do this is to gently push part of a 2 x 2 into the defect, leaving a portion of it outside for easy removal later. This allows the incision stay open longer, giving the body extra time to push out the remaining dead and infected material.

Even small collections can cause quite a bit of disability. Paronychia is an infection that occurs around the fingernail. The typical treatment is to soak it in warm water two or three times a day, but this rarely works.

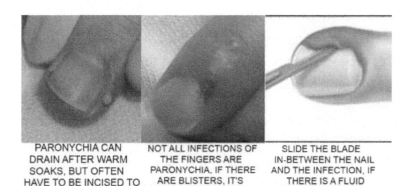

PARONYCHIA CAN DRAIN AFTER WARM SOAKS, BUT OFTEN HAVE TO BE INCISED TO COMPLETELY RESOLVE	NOT ALL INFECTIONS OF THE FINGERS ARE PARONYCHIA, IF THERE ARE BLISTERS, IT'S PROBABLY HERPETIC WHITLOW - DON'T INCISE!	SLIDE THE BLADE IN-BETWEEN THE NAIL AND THE INFECTION, IF THERE IS A FLUID COLLECTION, IT WILL DRAIN IN MOST CASES

In this condition, do not incise the skin like you would with an abscess. Instead slide the blade on top of the nail and under the skin. There is an invisible plane between these two structures, and once the blade is slipped into it, the puss collection will rush out. No drain is needed, but antibiotics may help if you fell it's not improving quickly enough.

Paronychia often results from unconscious nail biting. If it happens repeatedly, soaking fingers in bleach for a few minutes in the morning can help the person take note and stop the behavior.

Wounds and abscesses heal from the inside out, filling themselves in with new healthy tissue over time. This process is called granulation, and the larger the wound, the longer it takes.

While it's not pleasant to think about, the smell of a drained abscess can often tell you how dangerous the bacteria are. Those smelling the worse are often infected with anaerobic bacteria, an aggressive germ. In this case if you have antibiotics, use them. Also keep the wound open with a drain as you normally would for a large cavity.

Anaerobic bacteria aren't typically a problem for superficial skin infections, or abscesses occurring on the trunk or upper extremities. Those will usually be just fine by simply putting in a drain. Abscesses that occur on the lower half of the body have a greater tendency to harbor more aggressive germs. They often come from the colon, and as you shower, they wash down toward your feet and setup shop on the skin of your lower extremities.

You don't have to buy drains for your medical kit. Make one when you need it by cutting off one of the fingers of a rubber glove.

I prefer using a rubber drain to packing gauze inside a wound.   Gauze must be changed every 1-2 days and the procedure can be painful, but drains only need removing once.   So many physicians use them as a matter of routine.

While you can easily buy a variety for your kit, it's easiest just to make one when you need it.   All you have to do is to take an exam glove and cut off one of the fingers. Then cut the other end so this flat but tubular structure is open at both ends.   Fluid doesn't drain through the center like it would in a pipe, but instead creeps along the edges of the latex by a mechanism called capillary action.

Position most of the rubber material inside the abscess cavity, leaving only a half inch or so protruding from the wound.   Then run a single suture through both the drain and one of the skin edges and tie it to keep it from falling out.   *Never suture it to both sides of the cavity.* Doing that will effectively close the wound you're trying to keep open.

ANIMAL BITES

Other common and important injuries are bite wounds. When occurring on the hand they can be devastating.

Human bites are the most dangerous of any animal, save sharks and tigers... possibly bears.

When caused by a cat or snake, they're essentially puncture wounds, *and should never be closed*. If anything you may want to open them a little wider with your scalpel.

Dog bites result in more of a laceration than a puncture, but also need to be left open. Neither cat nor dog bites are as dangerous as those from people. The mouths of dogs and cats are much cleaner than ours. In all cases: cat, dog, or human, leave the wound open, irrigate with antiseptic solution, and treat with antibiotics if available. If it's a zombie bite, treat with a .45 slug to the noggin, and call it a day.

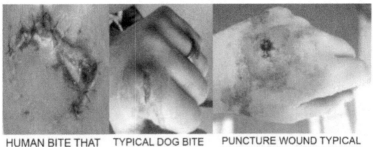

HUMAN BITE THAT SOMEONE TRIED TO CLOSE - NEVER DO THIS!!!

TYPICAL DOG BITE WOUND. BECAUSE IT LOOKS LIKE A LACERATION, IT'S CLOSED IN ERROR

PUNCTURE WOUND TYPICAL OF A CAT BITE. DON'T CLOSE. IF VERY SMALL AND NARROW, YOU MAY EVEN NEED TO OPEN IT UP SOME SO IT CAN DRAIN.

When you find yourself draining abscesses, take extra time to numb the skin before cutting. This can be difficult, particularly if the area is really inflamed. Infections cause acidity to build up in the skin, and can partially inactivate injectable anesthetics. So if you are injecting Lidocaine or Novocaine, you'll have much more than usual, and wait longer for it to take effect.

Sometimes people will get a fever when they have an abscess. Once drained, it should resolve. A person only has a fever if their temperature exceeds 100.4 degrees Fahrenheit. Fever may be a sign that the infection is spreading, and so it's a good idea to get a thermometer for your medical bag.

Human body temperature often fluctuates between 98 and 100 degrees. 100.4 degrees or more is considered a fever, but should not always be treated.

Try *not to treat a fever* with Tylenol, Aspirin, or Ibuprofen unless you have to.   The body naturally wants to warm itself when fighting an infection.   Increasing core temperature aids the immune system in killing the invading bacteria.

Nowadays, many doctors don't treat fevers unless they're causing discomfort.   This general rule holds true until the person's temperatures reaches 104 or more.   Then they'll treat.   But for a run of the mill infection, like the common cold, don't treat the fever if you can help it.   It's Nature's built-in antibiotic, and she's had phenomenal success with it despite our "common sense" view to the contrary.

SUGAR

It seems counterintuitive, but one way to control a wound infection is to fill the cavity with sugar, or better yet, with honey.   Everyone knows that bacteria replicate faster when supplied with a sugar source, but in its granulated form, sugar's concentration is so high it destroys microbes.

One of the most valuable outdoor skills a prepper can learn, is to build and use a bee smoker for collecting honey.

Honey is often more accessible in the field, and we discuss its antimicrobial properties and uses in more detail later.

These treatments have been used for centuries, and are still the standard of care in some parts of the world. This is one reason you'll want to find and collect sugar packets.   If you're putting together a medical kit, grab a few packs from the next restaurant you visit, and throw them into a Ziploc bag for later.

Cholesterol filled breakfasts may help save your life one day after all!

LACERATIONS & SKIN INJURIES — ANESTHESIA & IRRIGATION

Did you know that it was a Dentist that discovered anesthesia? That's bit of irony. But it has made life much easier in other venues.

Learning how to repair skin lacerations is easier than it used to be. YouTube videos and wikiHow pages can help. It's not as complicated as it looks. You try to keep the skin edges flat or slightly curved outward as you suture them together. Remember to wash out the wound before closing it, and leave a drain in if you think it might become infected.

If the wound is reasonably clean, I recommend injecting lidocaine into the skin margins before starting your irrigation. You'll be controlling pain from all stages of the repair better this way.

DRUG INTERACTIONS

We'll be discussing the use of injectable anesthetics next, but first we must talk about situations when they cannot be used.

There's a little known category of medications called monoamine oxidase inhibitors (MAOI's.)   Not a lot of people are taking them.   In the past they were prescribed for the treatment of psychiatric disorders that didn't respond to any other known medicines.   Nowadays, they're mostly used for the treatment of Parkinson's disease.   Pain medications like Demerol, and all injectable anesthetics, mustn't be used in people taking MAOI's.   The resulting drug interaction is often fatal.

Most people on these medications know about this interaction, and have been trained to tell a doctor that they're taking them.   But in times of stress they can forget, so you must always ask.   Selegiline and moclobemide are the names of two common examples.

Anti-nausea medications like Phenergan, Compazine, and others belonging to the phenothiazine family, can also cause this type of reaction.   Though they do so less often. So don't use injectable anesthetics unless you're sure the person you are about to inject isn't taking any of these medications.   And never perform any medical procedures if help is or will be available.

Injectable Anesthetics

Lidocaine and Xylocaine are the most popular injectable anesthetics.   Concentrations of 0.5%, 1% and 2%, with or without epinephrine are most common.   Stick with the 1%, and avoid mixtures containing epinephrine for now. Epinephrine constricts blood vessels, and is sometimes added to help control bleeding from wounds edges. Problems arise when the tissue being injected is fed by only one blood supply. Should that lone feeder vessel be closed off, you can end up killing all the surrounding tissue. Medical students remember the areas where anesthetic with epinephrine cannot be used by the rhyme: Fingers, nose, hose (penis), lobes (ear lobes) and toes.

> *Remember the Novocaine nursery rhyme: "No fingers, nose, hose, toes, or lobes."*

You can tell quickly if the Xylocaine you're using has epinephrine mixed in. The bottle label will be red and white. Plain lidocaine vials have blue and white or black and white printing.

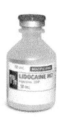 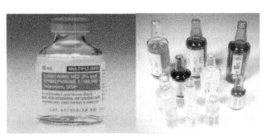

Lidocaine and Xylocaine are the same anesthetic. W/O added epinephrine is shown above.

2% lidocine with epinephrine. Note the red vs. blue label. Try to stay away from 2% concentration for now.

Single use ampules. Be sure you know how to open these. Otherwise you'll cut your hand or finger.

Lidocaine can be ordered on the internet, the Chinese sites appear to be the cheapest. Some people prefer to buy single use ampules instead of multi-dose vials. Some people are allergic to the preservatives added into the multi-dose vials, though in recent years many companies are removing it or changing to something less allergenic. This probably doesn't apply to lidocaine made outside of the country. So beware.

Procaine (Novocaine)

- o Novocaine was America's principle anesthetic for years, but eventually was replaced by lidocaine. It's dosed like lidocaine, and has many of the same characteristics.
- o It's short-acting and has extremely low toxicity.
- o Can usually be used for people allergic to lidocaine.

Lidocaine (Xylocaine)

- o Comes in 0.5%, 1 %, 2% concentrations; the maximum dose is 300mg (4mg/kg; 30ml of 1 %) and 500mg (7mg/kg; 50ml of 1 %) when mixed with epinephrine.
- o The onset is almost immediate with infiltration. It usually lasts an hour with 0.5% (2 hours with epinephrine) and 1.5 hours with 1 % (3.5 hours with epinephrine).

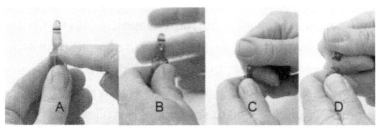

On the neck of the ampule, you will find a mark, usually a dot where the glass has been scored (A.) Tap any fluid lodged in the top out before breaking (B.) Put your index fingers firmly together (C) and rotate your right hand downward (D.)

Marcaine, a.k.a. Bupivacaine, is another useful anesthetic you'll want to become familiar with.   It takes longer to take effect, but lasts for six hours.

Bupivacaine (Marcaine)

- o Comes in 0.25% and 0.5% concentrations with a maximum of 175mg (70mL of 0.25%) when mixed with epinephrine. Not to be repeated within 3 hours with maximum 8mg/kg in 24 hours.
- o Has a slow onset of action, taking 10-20 minutes to take effect. However it lasts for 4 to 6 hours. It can be mixed with lidocaine (half lidocaine and half bupivacaine) to produce an anesthetic that starts acting quickly, and lasts up to 6 hours.

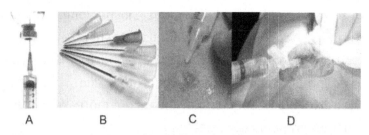

A   B   C   D

DRAW UP THE LIDOCAINE AFTER WIPING THE TOP OF THE VIAL WITH ALCOHOL (A). USE A LARGE NEEDLE, LIKE THE ONE ON THE BOTTOM, TO DRAW UP THE ANESTHETIC, AND A SMALL ONE, LIKE THE ONE ON TOP, TO INJECT IT (B). INJECT A "WHEEL" OF THE AGENT AROUND AN ABSCESS (C) OR INTO SKIN MARGINS OF A LACERATION (D) - NEVER REUSE NEEDLES!

Remember a few key points before you start drawing up the anesthetic. First, the needle used to pull out the Xylocaine will become increasingly dull each time it pierces through the vials rubber stopper. Second, you must not put the needle back into the bottle after it's been used to inject the patient, it will contaminate the remaining lidocaine. It's best to have a large bore needle for drawing up the anesthetic, and replace it with a small bore for injecting it. Repeat needle swapping as often as necessary, being careful not to confuse the two.

In health care, we never recap a needle after use. We dispose of it in a special container for sharp objects. Recapping increases the possibility of getting stuck with a contaminated needle. In the field, disposing of every needle after use may not be practical, not when there's a shortage of supplies.

I knew a Russian physician who told me of an experience he had in the Soviet Union during the 1980s. His entire hospital had only one hypodermic needle. It was an 18 gauge, and started off being 1 ½ inches long.   It would dull quickly, and frequently needed sharpening.   Eventually it was whittled down to about ¼ of an inch in length, and could no longer penetrate under the skin.   His story illustrates the reality of having to do more with less, a situation preppers can relate with.

USING ANESTHETICS

Typically you'll have to wait about five minutes before an anesthetic takes effect.   When preparing a laceration for repair, inject underneath the skin edges where the wound is open.   By avoiding a needle stick through intact skin, you save the patient discomfort and decrease the risk of infection.

Here is our short covering the common types of anesthetics, how to draw them up into a syringe, and how to inject them into a wound.

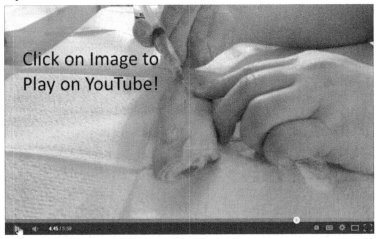

Click on Image to Play on YouTube!

https://www.youtube.com/watch?v=14lv9zlK78o

1% lidocaine without epinephrine is the type you'll want to keep in your bag if you plan to suture wounds. It can be used for most repairs and procedures, including draining abscesses.

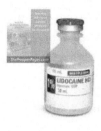 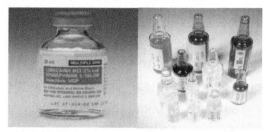

Lidocaine and Xylocaine are the same anesthetic. W/O added epinephrine is shown above.	2% lidocine with epinephrine. Note the red vs. blue label. Try to stay away from 2% concentration for now.	Single use ampules. Be sure you know how to open these. Otherwise you'll cut your hand or finger.

TRICKS WE'VE LEARNED FROM DENTISTS

Have you ever had the dentist wiggle your cheek a bit while giving you a shot of Novocaine? It helps with the injection pain quite a bit. It works by piggybacking onto, and then overloading the nerves carrying pain signals. You can use this trick by moving the persons skin back and forth quickly near the wound you're about to repair. Pain fibers will become "confused" and lose some of their ability to transmit painful sensations. The technique is especially useful when you don't have lidocaine, and can only put ice on the skin for a while beforehand. The ice trick works reasonably well in decreasing the person's pain as the needle is entering into their skin.

DIGITAL NERVE BLOCKS — NUMBING FINGERS & TOES

By blocking the entire digit from pain, you make it much easier to clean and subsequently close a wound. There isn't much extra skin on fingers, so if you were to decide to inject into the wound margins, you'd be causing some degree of tissue swelling as the medicine enters. The edges might not come together as well as you'd wish.

A digital block avoids this problem by injecting lidocaine into the web spaces on each side of the finger, instead of along the cut skin margins.   It's much easier to perform than you may think, and practicing on a pig's foot first will provide you all the confidence you'll need.   We'd like to show you how that's done in the following video:

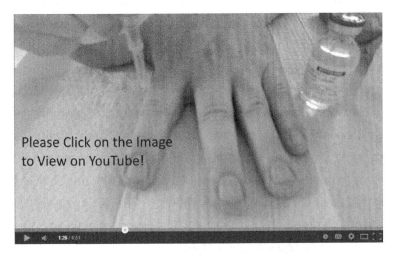

Please Click on the Image to View on YouTube!

https://www.youtube.com/watch?v=BuBf4bpL4Zs

The procedure involves injecting lidocaine into the web spaces on either side of the finger or toe you're numbing. By blocking the nerves as they exit the area on their way to the finger tip, you deaden the entire digit. Five minutes are usually required before the analgesic effect makes its way from the web space to the fingertip.

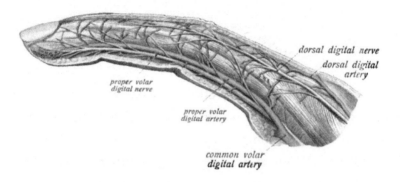

dorsal digital nerve

dorsal digital artery

proper volar digital nerve

proper volar digital artery

common volar digital artery

Some parts of the body have only one vessel providing fresh oxygenation to distal tissues. Fingers and toes are a good example. Lidocaine can be used to numb these areas, but only if it does not contain epinephrine. Epinephrine shuts off the blood supply to the area, so if you inject it into a finger or toe, you'll completely shut off its only avenue of oxygenation. The tissue will become gangrenous, and the person will lose their finger.

For this technique you'll want to use 1%, or preferably 2% lidocaine *without* epinephrine. Recall that a lidocaine bottle with a red label means the mixture contains epinephrine. A blue or black label means it's free of this component, and can safely be used for the digital block procedure.

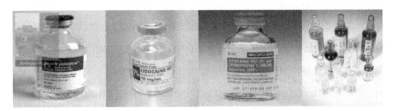

XYLOCAINE AND LIDOCAINE ARE THE SAME TYPE OF MEDICATION.
BOTH COME IN DIFFERENT STRENGTHS, AND IN SINGLE USE AND
MULTIPLE DOSE VIALS. IF YOU HAVE A CHOICE, USE THE 1%.
LIDOCAINE WITH EPINEPHRINE IS FOR SPECIAL USE AND COMES
IN A BOTTLE WITH A RED LABEL. THE FAR RIGHT PICTURE SHOWS
A VARIETY OF AMPULES, ANOTHER FORM LIDOCAINE COMES IN.

We recommend injecting the web space through the back of the hand, as the palmar side is rich in nerve fibers and hurts more when punctured.   Fill a syringe with 3 ml's of 1% or 2% lidocaine without epinephrine.   You'll be injecting half that amount (1-1.5 ml's) on each side of the finger.   Remember to lightly scrub the skin with an alcohol swab before inserting the needle.

Begin by squeezing the tissue of your patient's web space between the index finger and thumb of your left hand. This helps create space between the skin and bone.   You don't want to hit the bone with your needle – *it's painful if you do*.   You might want to place ice on the skin over the spot you plan to inject for 60-90 seconds right before.   It will decrease the person's discomfort as the needle is penetrating through their skin.

Once you're in, carefully advance the needle straight down toward the skin on the palmar side.   Don't let it travel all the way down and puncture through the other side.

You'll feel the skin on the palmar side start to tent as you get close.

Now, slowly withdraw the needle back out, injecting lidocaine at a constant rate as you do.   Go slow.   By the time you get back up to the place where you started from, your injection on that side will be complete.

Repeat the procedure on the other side of the same digit.   Again delivering 1-1.5 ml's of anesthetic as you're slowly backing the needle out.   It takes a little work to get the coordination right.   After practicing on a pig's foot a couple of times, it will become much easier.   If you want the finger to stay numb longer than two hours, add Marcaine to the mix.   Please see the appendix for further instructions.

WHAT IF YOU DON'T HAVE LIDOCAINE?

You may not have access to local anesthetics, but still need to sew up a laceration.   What can you do?

Use the ice trick.   Hold an ice cube on the laceration for two minutes, then quickly remove it and sneak in in one of your stitches.   This works much better than you'd think. The point to keep in mind, is to stop after each stitch and reapply the ice.

Remember this technique, it will get you through when your supplies were limited.   Having used it on myself twice, I estimate it reduces the pain by 80%.

Try to inject enough anesthetic to make the wound edges bevel upward as they fill with fluid. You'll find this aids in the repair, and ensures you've placed enough anesthetic into the skin margins.

About five minutes after injecting, grasp the skin with forceps to make sure it's numb. If it's not completely deadened, either wait a few more minutes, or inject more anesthetic.

There is a limit to how much you can safely use. It varies with the anesthetic and its concentration. When injecting 1% lidocaine, don't use more than 3 ml per kilogram of the person's body weight. But reaching the maximum dose is rarely an important consideration. If a patient weighs 70 kg, then the upper limit you can safely inject is 210 ml's. An average laceration shouldn't require more than about 10 ml's.

CLEANING WOUNDS - "IRRIGATION"

When the wound is numb, start your irrigation. Draw up some sterile water or saline into a large syringe. If you have one, hook up an 18 gauge intravenous catheter sleeve to your syringe and start washing debris out of the wound. Repeat filling and emptying the syringe into the wound until it's been thoroughly cleaned.

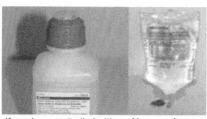 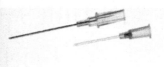

		In a controlled environment like an
If you have a sterile bottle of saline, you don't have to use a syringe for irrigation. Poke holes in the top with an 18 gauge needle. Turn upside down and squeeze like a spray nozzle to wash.	You can draw sterile saline out of an IV bag, or put an 18 gauge needle into the port on the right and squeeze.	aid station, you may prefer using a IV catheter shown above.

In the field, the two methods shown on the left seem to work the best. They take the least amout of time and preparation. |

Ideally you'll want to use 500 ml irrigation, but this is rarely practical.   Just wash until the all of the foreign debris has been removed, that's about the best you can do.

For added antimicrobial effect, try adding some hydrogen peroxide or Betadine to the saline.   Sterile water or saline can be difficult to come by.   But even using plain tap water has been shown to reduce infection rates. Mixed with Betadine, it probably doesn't matter if the fluid is sterile, just clean.

Here comes the really fun part - putting in stitches!

Lacerations & Skin Injuries – Stitches & Equipment

Does stitching someone back together seem intimidating? How about doing a Rambo and sewing your own skin shut? After the next few chapters the mystery and magic will dissolve, as will your anxiety. You might even want to learn more advanced methods, so I've put a few of the most valuable in the appendices. But here's how to start:

After cleaning the wound replace your gloves with a clean pair. If using sterile technique, put on an individually wrapped sterile pair.

Performing strictly sterile procedures is beyond the scope of this manual, but is easily learned from instructional videos if you're interested. Sterile technique should be used whenever possible. But in our theater of operation, being "germ free" is wishful thinking. In certain areas, like lacerations of the scalp, it's not even possible.

Start the repair by placing the semi-circular needle into the needle holder or "needle driver."

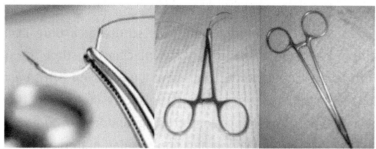

THIS INSTRUMENT WON'T WORK AS A NEEDLE HOLDER THE NEEDLE WILL ROLL!

THE JAWS SHOULD NOT BE SERRATED BUT FLAT

USE STRAIT AND FLAT JAWED NEEDLE HOLDERS - AVOID THE CURVED ONES

Needle drivers have smooth or lightly textured jaws, and may look like hemostats. Hemostats differ though in having large serrations resembling teeth. If you're going to buy a needle driver, I suggest getting one with built-in scissors.

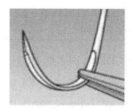 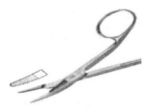

TO BEGIN, GRASP THE SUTURE NEEDLE WITH THE DRIVER ABOUT 2/3rds DOWN ITS LENGTH (LEFT). NEEDLE DRIVERS CAN HAVE SMOOTH OR TEXTURED JAWS, BUT NOT TEETH (CENTER). TEETH INDICATE THE INSTRUMENT IS A HEMO-STAT. DRIVERS WITH SCISSORS BUILT IN ARE THE MOST EASY TO USE (RIGHT).

Available in four and six inch sizes, they're easy to use and save time. The four inch is best for small cuts, six inch for large gashes.

GETTING STARTED

We recommend placing one suture at a time in a simple interrupted fashion. After placing the stitch, tie it with several square knots to prevent it unraveling. It's best to leave a long tail when cutting the suture material. This also prevents the knot from coming undone, a common problem when using nylon and non-braided materials.

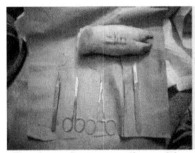

Begin suture practice with a pig's foot or chicken leg.

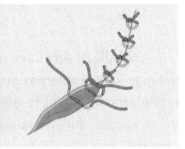

Simple interrupted sutures allow you to open just part of the wound if it gets infected.

Many people march down the laceration, placing one suture at a time until the wound is closed. But there's a more exact method. It's called the rule of halves, and it ensures the spacing will be correct.

RULE OF HALVES

When putting in individual stitches, follow the rule of halves. The rule states the first stitch should be placed in the center of the laceration, and later stitches should divide the remaining space into two areas of equal size. Continue dividing either side into equal spaces with each new stitch.

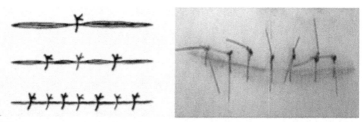

Simple interrupted sutures are easiest to place when using the rule of halves. The suture material shown on the right is made of non-braided nylon. Note the long tails and multiple knots keeping it from unraveling.

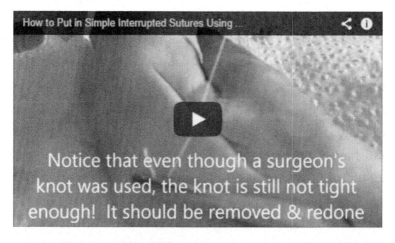

How to Put in Simple Interrupted Sutures Using ...

Notice that even though a surgeon's knot was used, the knot is still not tight enough! It should be removed & redone

Placing simple interrupted sutures is the preferred method, because if the wound becomes infected, you can remove every other suture and let it drain while still keeping the laceration edges approximated.   This is impossible if you run your stitch.

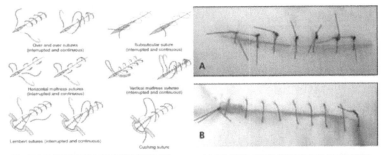

THERE ARE MANY DIFFERENT
TYPES OF SUTURE TECHNIQUES
STAY WITH SIMPLE OR RUNNING

A) SIMPLE INTERRUPTED SUTURES
B) RUNNING SUTURE - EASY BUT
CAN EASILY COME UNDONE

Practice suturing with pig's feet or chicken drumsticks. Medical students have learned this way for years. In little time you can become proficient. Another strategy is to bring together a bunch of interested people and have someone come in and teach the group. In a couple of hours you'll become confident in your skills and even learn advanced techniques. Suturing is one of the most satisfying emergency skills you can learn. Basic techniques are outlined in this and upcoming chapters. Advanced skills are illustrated in the appendix.

Pig's feet have been used for years in suturing practice.

Start by learning to place simple interrupted sutures, then move on to running and mattress techniques.

Check the appendix for details on performing advanced skills.

You might find it tempting to give oral antibiotics after the wound has been closed to prevent infections. But studies have shown giving oral antibiotics in this setting actually *increases* the risk of infection. Both helpful and harmful bacteria live on your skin. The helpful ones compete for living space with the harmful forms. Unfortunately, helpful bacteria are the ones most susceptible to antibiotics. They get killed off and are unable to help prevent the bad bacteria from causing infections.

Antibiotic prophylaxis should be avoided for most potential infections. Start them only when you clearly see an infection has developed. Otherwise they're too valuable to waste, and are probably more harmful than helpful.

Most lacerations will heal in seven to ten days. You can remove the sutures earlier if you need to, but the earlier you remove them, the greater the chance the wound will reopen.

Don't leave them in too long, or you might get an infection from the suture itself. The person may also get a larger scar, but this is not a major concern after the fall of civilization.

SUTURE REMOVAL

Timing of Suture Removal

Suture Location	Days until removal
Face	3-5
Scalp	7-10
Trunk	7-10
Arms/legs	10-14
Fingertips	10-12
Palms/soles	14

The closer the wound is to the heart, the faster it heals. This means that a laceration occurring on the hand will heal more slowly than one on the upper arm. Consequently, the hand sutures will need to be left in longer.

Sometimes they can be difficult to get out. They get caught up in the scab formation. See the appendix for instructions on the removal process.

CONCENTRATED LIDOCAINE WITH AND WITHOUT EPINEPHRINE

Avoid using lidocaine in concentrations greater than 1% unless you're performing a digital block.

When mixed with epinephrine, the anesthetic can be used for more than laceration repairs. To treat nose bleeds, squirt lidocaine with epinephrine on a 2 x2, roll it up tightly, and insert it into the bleeding nostril. This will help constrict the blood vessels and stop the bleeding.

Just a few more considerations, then we're off to the really juicy stuff!

HANDLING FLESH

BLEEDING CONTROL

For any wound the bleeding must be controlled. Apply direct pressure for several minutes, often that's all needed. Head and facial wounds tend to bleed most heavily. Always wear gloves and protective eye wear. DO NOT get someone else's blood borne infection.

LOCATION

Facial wounds are cosmetically noticeable, and need meticulous handling to decrease scar formation. Wounds over joints are under tension. Protect the repair with splints or other devices to prevent tugging that might cause the stitches to pull through. While minimum scarring is desired, scar formation on the torso or extremities is more acceptable than on the face. Select very fine material for closing facial cuts, and take the sutures out as soon as possible.

INITIAL TISSUE HANDLING

Wound appearance after healing is influenced by many factors. The age and race of the patient, the mechanism and location of the wound, and the patient's inherent ability to heal are important considerations.

Excessive scar formation can be minimized by gentle handling of the tissue, and careful but thorough cleansing of the wound.

In the past it was thought that wounds should be closed within twelve hours of occurrence. And facial wounds within 24 hours. This timeframe is referred to as the "golden period," after which a wound should not be sutured shut. But studies show this no longer applicable. Most wounds, even those days old, can be repaired if they're not infected.

There are Inventive ways to avoid suturing all together. One was stolen from the Soviets during their fall, the other from our own pilots during WWII. Let's see what happened:

SUPER-GLUING AMERICANS & STAPLING SOVIETS

I often wish the 80s never ended. It wasn't much different than the 70s I imagine, other than the clothes got even worse. But as the 80s closed, and the wall fell, the Soviets opened their libraries to the world.

Suspecting there were hidden gems in their technology vaults, Western Pharmaceutical Companies sent their scientific sleuths over to the Russian Federation to see what they could dig up.

Before long they unearthed plans for a stapling device. One that could quickly reattach two ends of cut intestine back together, and required few steps. Best of all, the process would only take about a minute. But there was a problem…

The Soviets couldn't get it to work.

But the Germans could. And did! The plans were copied and taken back to Germany and the United States, where the design was perfected and the rest is history. It was one of the greatest advances in surgery of the 20th century.

That same technology was dummied down and simplified for use on the skin. Cutaneous skin staplers are now widely used. They offer an alternative to placing stitches on the scalp and extremities.

Cutaneous skin staplers are widely used in surgery and emergency medicine, and offer a quick alternative to stitches. Their use is avoided on the face, and is generally reserved for wounds of the scalp, trunk, and extremities. Available from a number of sources, they generally run $15-30.

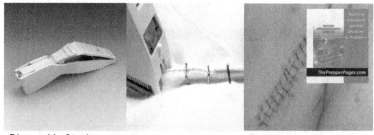

Disposable Staplers are not reloadable, but they have gotten smaller and less expensive

Practice placing skin staples on a bed sheet- See the YouTube video: http://youtu.be/uzpswG 7UXME

Remove the skin staples when you would remove stitches. The timing of both is the same

The drawback is the device only holds 15-30 staples, and is not reloadable. A staple removal instrument is also required, and must be purchased separately. This being so, they can still save you a lot of time and avoid having to learn suturing techniques.

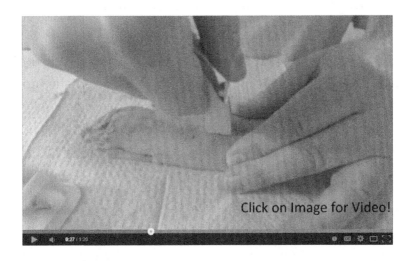

Click on Image for Video!

https://www.youtube.com/watch?v=uzpswG7UXME

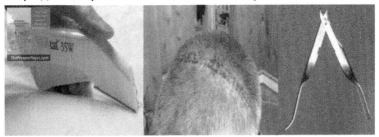

Skin staplers make laceration repair quick and easy, but are expensive. They can't be reloaded and generally come with 25 staples. Another drawback is that you must have a staple remover, they don't come with the device & must be purchased seperately.

SUPERGLUE

During WW II, pilots often had broken shards of their clear acrylic canopy implant in their arms and face. This shrapnel was produced by bullets tearing through the cockpit. Frequently, these embedded acrylic pieces were never found or removed.

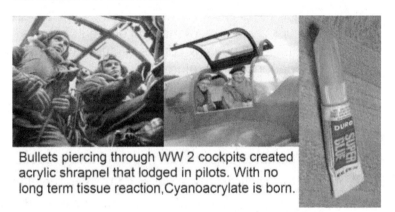

Bullets piercing through WW 2 cockpits created acrylic shrapnel that lodged in pilots. With no long term tissue reaction,Cyanoacrylate is born.

Years later the Veterans Administration noticed the fragments were not dissolving or festering out. The body was not reacting to them at all. This finding paved the way to using acrylic based adhesives to close small and medium sized wounds.

Super glue is very similar in molecular structure to surgical adhesives. You can save a lot of time and hassle by using one of these liquid acrylics to repair lacerations. Dermabond is one such product (shown in the picture below).

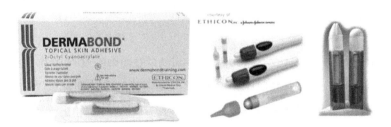

There are several versions of medical grade superglue
Dermabond is best known & comes in different forms
In our experience superglue works just as well!

Purchasing surgical adhesive isn't always necessary. You can use super glue, or crazy glue as an acceptable substitute. The advantage that Dermabond and products like it offer, is the applicators are designed to keep the glue on the skin and out of the wound. Crazy glue takes a little more finesse to apply correctly.

When can super glue be used in place of stitches?

Whenever you feel the wound you're closing has minimal tension on the edges as you pinch them together. That's the first criteria.

The second, is you must be able to keep the super glue from pouring into the wound. If it does, it will prevent the edges from touching. If anything comes between these cut skin margins, they won't seal back together correctly. If you can meet these requirement, then you can use super glue instead of sutures to close the laceration.

Tip: *The trick is to keep the glue on the skin, and not let any of it get into the wound. If this happens, super glue won't work. Stitches will be required. Otherwise the laceration will just pull apart later.*

This brings us to our next challenge. How do you suture or staple a wound back together on the world's most skittish animal? Yes... *I'm talking about those little critters called children!*

TREATING INJURIES IN CHILDREN & OTHER WILD ANIMALS

No matter how you look at it, children are tough customers. And when it comes to sewing them up, it's best to give the sedative to yourself first.

Physicians have a few tricks for dealing with these little fighters. Playing "mummy" is one of our favorite!

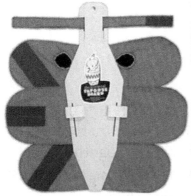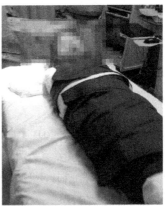

A papoose board is found in nearly every hospital ER in the United States. You probably won't have one of these, so with bedsheets & tape, you'll need to play the game "mummy".

Sometimes we'll place the child on a Papoose Board. It constrains the movement of their body and head, allowing us to complete the repair. But more often than not, we can't find the board when we need it. And in the field zombie preppers surely won't be packing one around.

So what can you do?

A bed sheet wrapped tightly around the child, with the arms tucked securely inside, will constrain the little monster nicely. Reinforce it with tape and secure them to a treatment table, and you'll be good to go!

The trick of course is to begin the game "let's play mummy" long before they learn they're about to get stitches. Otherwise you're in for nothing but pure drama. It's easier to get your cat to jump in the car for his neutering appointment, than it is to find a child that's just heard the word "stitches."

Start the game by having the child put their arms to their sides, then start wrapping. When you're done, reinforce the costume with tape all the way around the chest, arms, and legs. You'll probably be repairing a forehead laceration; kids seem to sustain injury there the most. Taping their head to the table is usually also required. Even with all of this, you'll still be working on a moving target to some degree.

After the child is done screaming and fighting, and you're done with the repair, expect them to suddenly fall asleep.   This doesn't mean they have a head injury or concussion, only that they're thoroughly exhausted.

Finally, one obvious but often forgotten trick.   Inject additional lidocaine just as you're about to finish - *before the initial injection wears off.*   If the repair is taking longer than expected, or if you want the analgesia to last a few hours after you're finished, inject them now while they still can't feel it.

Now with the basics of wound closure complete, let's tackle the most miserable of aliments encountered in the field:

BURNS

Burns are some of the most grotesque and brutal injuries of war and cataclysms. They're classified by the number of layers of tissue they involve. First, second, and third degree burns are referred to most commonly. The term "fourth degree" is sometimes used for those involving the underlying bone.

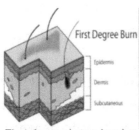

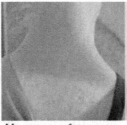

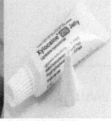

First degree burns involve the epidermis or outer layer only. They can be quite painful, but don't result in large fluid losses.

Many occur from sunburns, hot radiators, stoves, or engines.

Lidocaine jelly works well for pain control, but has to be applied every couple of hours.

FIRST DEGREE BURNS

The first layer of skin is called the epidermis, and it's rich with underlying pain receptors. Burns here are confined to the outer layer of skin, though they often peel or blister later. They're harmful in the sense that the pain they cause, can be incapacitating. Severe sunburns can limit a person's ability to travel, and carry their supplies.

Treating the pain with lidocaine gel, which comes in 2% and 4% concentrations, is controversial. It's normally used for numbing the skin prior to laceration repair or complicated injections. But it can be smeared over the most sensitive burns to keep a person mobile.

Baking soda in water, and witch hazel, both draw heat and the sensation it produces out of wounds.

While not approved or even recommend for sunburns, I've found lidocaine gel helpful. If a prepper needs it to stay mobile to trek to safety, it might be worth the small risk. Studies have not been done to find out how much of the gel can be safely used before person becomes toxic. It probably shouldn't be used on children for this reason. If you don't have the gel, you can make some. Draw 5-10 ml's of lidocaine from your multi-dose vial and mix it into an ointment or cortisone cream. Again this isn't recommended or even approved by the FDA. I've experimented with putting injectable lidocaine into a spray bottle, and delivering it that way. But the relief only lasts for 20 – 30 minutes, then reapplication is needed. In mixing my own lidocaine 1% for injection with a cream, or putting it in a spray bottle, I wasn't worried about an overdose. A multi-use vial only has 50 ml's in it. That's only a fraction of the 210 ml's marking the ceiling.

For children and adults, you can apply strips of cloth soaked in cold water to the burns. Mixed with baking soda or cold witch hazel, this can help treat pain and slow fluid loss. Baking soda and witch hazel are both endothermic, meaning they provide pain relief by drawing out heat.

Cold water does this better, but not might be available without refrigeration. Use this treatment for all burns, it's another potential use of the bed sheets you've already cut into strips.

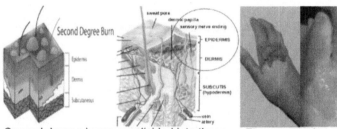

Second degree burns are divided into those superficial and those deep. Superficial burns are very painful, deep wounds are not. This is because in deep wounds, the nerve endings have been destroyed.

These wounds can both blister and weep. They can result in massive and fatal fluid loss when extensive.

SECOND DEGREE BURNS

Divided into two functional and anatomical classifications, second degree burns can be superficial, deep, or a combination of the two. Telling the difference relies on the symptoms they produce.

Superficial wounds are very painful. Deep burns aren't. Though they can produce the sensations of pressure and discomfort. Nerve endings conveying pain are essentially melted away in deep wounds, so typical pain signals aren't transmitted to the brain.

Large deep second degree burns cause massive fluid loss. Intravenous fluid replacement is required if they total more than 20% of the persons total body surface area (TBSA.) Burns involving 30-40% may be fatal without hospital treatment.

Burns must be covered with the cleanest dressings possible. Avoid repetitive examinations, they only increase the infection rate.

While there are formulas for calculating the effected TBSA, the easiest way to estimate it in the field is with the patient's hand. The area of their palm equals about 1% of their TBSA.

First degree burns are not calculated into the surface area estimation, only second and third degree.   If someone in your group has sustained injures to more than 30-40% of their body surface, they may not survive without conventional medical care.

Honey

KEEP AN EYE OUT FOR A BOTTLE OF HONEY WHILE YOU'RE ON THE MOVE.   IT'S A VERY EFFECTIVE TOPICAL ANTIBIOTIC THAT CAN BE USED FOR BURNS AND OTHER WOUNDS.

The best you can do in a situation like this, is to wrap them in moist strips of cloth, and throw pain medications at them.   Dehydration from large weeping wounds pose the primary threat.   Potentially lethal skin infections the secondary.   It's a bad scene all around.

If placed in the hospital, the person would probably be covered with silver sulfadiazine or silver nitrate solution, and silver-impregnated dressings.   Topical antibiotics purchased over the counter aren't capable of penetrating eschars, which are the hard inflexible scars that result from burns.   Silver based ointments and creams can, and are used in hospitals for this reason.

For the prepper it's impossible to carry enough silver sulfadiazine for this contingency. A single bottle for small burns may be useful, but for large injuries you'll need something you can find in the local environment. Studies show honey can fill this need and work as a clever substitute.

Honey has native antibacterial properties. This makes sense when you think about it, otherwise it wouldn't be able to survive the outdoors in a bee hive. Honey has also been shown to help debride wounds by removing the dead tissue. Anti-inflammatory properties, and the ability to stimulate the growth of granulation and epithelial tissue, have also been observed.

Use a tongue depressor to spread it over the burns, remembering to give the patient pain medication beforehand. As superficial and deep second degree injuries are usually mixed, the process of applying honey, or another topical treatment, can be painful.

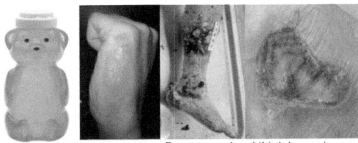

Honey is a multifunctional item. As with all topical antibiotics, it can be difficult to keep on the burn, like the one shown above.

Deep second and third degree burns form scars called eschars. They can harbor bacteria and serve as a source of infection. They must be cut away.

Like granular sugar, honey can also be used to treat abscess cavities, making it one of the most important items to look for as you're collecting supplies.

THIRD DEGREE BURNS

These penetrate down to the fat layer and sometimes bone.   Amputation is often required.   Keep the person as comfortable as possible and try to prevent infection by applying topical antibiotics or honey.

Multiple Uses for Popsicle

POPSICLE STICKS CAN SERVE AS TONGUE DEPRESSORS, LOOK FOR THEM WHILE ON THE MOVE. NEXT TIME YOU ARE AT YOUR DOCTOR'S OFFICE, ASK IF YOU CAN HAVE A FEW DEPRESSORS FOR YOUR KIT.

Burns are awful.   There is a painless way to debride them...but you're probably not going to like it!

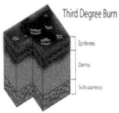 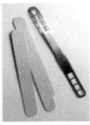 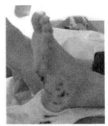

Third degree burns extend into the fat layer under the skin. Tongue depressors have many uses, from splinting fractures to applying topical creams. Ask your doctor for a few.

Popsicle sticks also work, and should be scavenged when possible. Electrical burns (far right) also form eschars, and can become infected.

In burn centers across the country, leeches are kept in a tank, either in the intensive care unit or in the pharmacy. The last ones I used I bought over the internet on Leechesusa.com. They're specially bred for medical use; meaning they've had all dangerous microorganisms removed.

Every day they're removed from the tank, applied to the patient's wounds, then collected and destroyed after falling off. You'll be able to find your own in swamps, though you can't be sure they aren't carrying some sort of disease. It's not a real big concern, because here leech borne diseases are very rare.

Put them in the burns, and let them feed until they fall off. Then put them back in your makeshift tank. I've done this myself. Once you get over the horror of it, you'll find they debride wounds much better, and less painfully, than you can do on your own.

Since we're on the topic of war injuries, let's talk about sword and musket ball wounds:

SHANKING & SHOTGUNNING – TREATING PROJECTILE WOUNDS

People often think if they get shot that it's imperative to remove the bullet.   After all, that's how it's done in the movies.   The real world works a bit differently.   Unless easily accessible, surgeons rarely remove bullets. Insistence on bullet removal has changed history a number of times.   For example, many modern surgeons feel that if President Lincoln's doctors wouldn't have tried removing his bullet (*eight times*), he'd probably survived his injury.

Digging around for foreign bodies often causes additional problems.   With regard to bullets, you won't get lead poisoning from leaving them in the body.   A tissue capsule forms around the projectile so the lead never seeps into your system.   Additionally, high velocity bullets are sterile when they exit the barrel, owing to the heat produced from the friction.   This wasn't the case back in the years of muskets and flintlocks.   But in today's world when infections develop, it's because bits of contaminated clothing have accompanied the projectile deep into the tissue.   So if you're going to remove anything, focus on finding the clothing shrapnel and forget the bullet fragments.

Smooth projectiles like bullets often don't need to be removed. Irregularly shaped projectiles and debris should be removed, as they harbor bacteria. Clothing and vegetation are the biggest culprits.

Organic projectiles - like flying pieces of wood - carry high infection rates. During WWII exploding trees from German artillery is thought to have caused more morbidity than the shrapnel itself.

Try to remove splinters of wood and any other *accessible* debris when possible. Then irrigate with copious amounts of antiseptic solution. Unless they are very superficial, and you're sure that all the debris has been retrieved, don't close these injuries like you would with a laceration. Leave them open and place a drain. With low velocity projectile injuries, that's about all you can do in the field.

Penetrating Abdominal Wounds

Gunshot and stab wounds of the abdomen are not inevitably fatal, despite the common perception. If a surgeon is not available, the best you can do is to give the person oral antibiotics, and limit food intake for a few days. Don't go digging. Sometimes penetrating bowel injuries will auto-seal. They probably do so more often than we think. Limit the person's activity and don't allow them to move around much.

That being said, no one should be completely immobilized. Everyone should move around a little, or they'll risk forming blood clots in their legs. Pieces of the clot can break off and travel to the lungs. When this happens, a pulmonary embolism results. They're rare, but can be more fatal than the wound itself. At minimum have them move their legs around several times a day.

People sustaining injuries to the intestine will sometimes develop something called a fistula. Inflammation from the injury will cause the bowel to adhere to the abdominal wall. When this happens, intestinal fluids and contents will start to seep out through the skin. This horrifies people, but it's the best thing that could happen. It means that those contents are not spilling inside the abdomen, and that the person is likely to survive.

<u>Side Note</u>: Can a Zombie Prepper Survive Appendicitis Without an Operation?

It's an important question for preppers. They know surgeons are going to be hard to find during prolonged disasters. So can a person survive appendicitis without an operation?

The problem confronted a lone surgeon stationed at a remote outpost in the South Pole years ago. He'd come down with appendicitis and decided to take his own out using mirrors and a couple of assistants. Ballsy for sure, but a little impractical for the rest of us.

WHAT IS APPENDICITIS?

No one is quite sure what the appendix is for, let alone why we get appendicitis. But we do know when this hollow tube becomes obstructed, bacteria multiply and have no way of getting out. Consequently the appendix becomes inflamed, and as it swells, it progressively irritates the lining of the lower abdominal cavity.

Usually beginning with tenderness around the belly button, the pain slowly radiates to the lower right quadrant of the abdomen. From there it commonly spreads widely, until the person is tender from the rib cage down.

It's important to note that in most cases, the pain of appendicitis proceeds vomiting. If vomiting appears first, then it's much less likely the person has appendicitis.

The classic symptoms of appendicitis:
Usually beginning as a dull discomfort near the navel, the pain becomes sharp as it moves to the lower right abdomen.
Loss of appetite
Nausea and/or vomiting soon after abdominal pain begins
Low Grade Fever of 100.4-102 degrees F
Pain that precedes vomiting

As the disease progresses, the entire abdomen becomes rigid and tender. Traveling over bumps in a car, or simply tapping on the person's heel with your fist when their leg is straightened, produces severe pain in the abdomen.

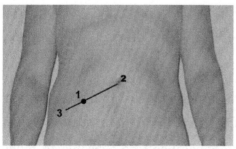

Pain often begins at location 2, then it travels to 1, where the appendix is found. From 1 it radiates everywhere.

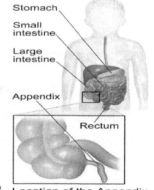

Location of the Appendix

TREATING APPENDICITIS WITH ORAL ANTIBIOTICS ONLY

(More information about antibiotics for zombie preppers will be coming up in our fish-i-cillin chapter a bit later in this book.)

Appendicitis may not always necessitate an operation. Data from nuclear submarines - which do not have surgeons on board - showed that 85% of sailors with suspected appendicitis recovered without surgery. But they were treated with intravenous antibiotics.

A much larger study involving 252 Swedish patients with appendicitis randomized them into two groups: one was treated with surgery, and the other with I.V. antibiotics. Of the 128 patients who did not undergo surgery, 88% recovered, and the other 12% eventually required operation.

In all of these studies intravenous antibiotics, not oral antibiotics, were used to treat the patients opting out of surgery. I.V. access probably won't be available to many preppers, and if it were, there are serious concerns about how fast those preparations go out of date. This means most preppers without surgical access will be relying on oral antibiotics alone. And while oral antibiotics might not be as effective as their intravenous counterparts, they are still effective and likely the best you can do in a nightmare scenario. So choosing the right oral antibiotics becomes important.

The I.V. equivalent to what has traditionally been used to treat appendicitis includes one antibiotic to kill anaerobic bacteria (species that do not need oxygen to live) and one to cover aerobic forms. Flagyl (Metronidazole) or Clindamycin are good choices for anaerobic species, and Augmentin (or similar Penicillin & Sulbactam combinations) take care of the aerobic bacteria.

Biology has an unbelievable ability to heal itself. Give the person every possible chance to get better. Despite our appearance, we're remarkably resilient creatures.

Now that you know what you're going to need in the field, let's talk about how to recycle your supplies:

FIELD STERILIZATION & SANITATION

Instruments can't be sterilized in the field, no matter what anyone says. But *sanitizing* needles, scalpels, and other essential equipment is possible. For instruments made of metal, the quickest and easiest method is to hold them over a flame. For needles, remember that the inside bore must be sanitized first.

Bleach & Its Concentration

AS YOU'RE RIFLING THROUGH A HOUSE, PAUSE IN THE LAUNDRY ROOM. ALMOST ALL CONTAIN BLEACH. POUR SOME INTO A SMALL CONTAINER. IF YOU CAN FIND ONE, USE A METAL THERMOS BOTTLE, THE TYPE THAT CAN BE USED TO BOIL WATER IN LATER.

Syringes and their pistons, needle bores, catheters, and other hollow items can be sanitized with alcohol or bleach solution. The alcohol should be 70% concentration or greater, and must be either isopropyl alcohol or ethanol (drinking alcohol) to be effective. Wood alcohol, regardless of its concentration, is useless. Bleach solution should be at least 5% concentrated, but only keeps for one year. To use either of these for sanitation, rinse one of these solutions through the syringes and needles, then let them soak for 30 - 40 minutes.

Bleach is a good substitute for Betadine. In the field, they're often interchangeable. So if you're rummaging for supplies, don't overlook the laundry room.

Trying to carry an entire gallon of bleach out into the field clearly won't work. Pour it into something smaller like a water bottle. Better yet, find a metal thermos cup with a no spill lid. You can use it later to boil water with. The newer models are much smaller than the silver bricks our parents carried to work. But be sure that whatever you transfer it into won't be mistaken for water by a thirsty child!

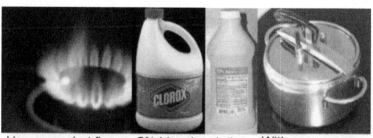

Use a very hot flame. Remember to first clean the bore of the syringe and needle.

5% bleach solution or 70% isopropyl or ethanol can be used to soak instruments.

With a pressure cooker, use 15 lbs. pressure for 15 minutes.

FIELD STERILIZATION AND SANITIZATION PROCEDURES

To make the bleach solution, pour ½ cup of undiluted bleach into 3 ½ cups of clean water. Dry the instruments before storing them.

Instruments can be sterilized once you've arrived at your bug-out location (BOL). This is easiest done with a pressure cooker set at 15 lbs. pressure for 15 minutes. Add five teaspoons of oil to the solution, it will help prevent rust.

If you want to keep equipment sterile after pressure cooking it, you'll have to put them in sterilizing packages beforehand. These are inexpensive and come in a variety of sizes. Always buy those bigger than you think you'll need. If you plan on using them directly after pressure cooking, then the packages aren't needed.

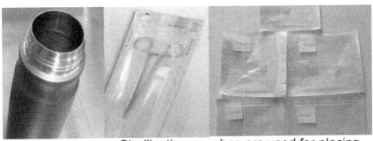

Thermos cups are great for boiling water and storing fluids in.

Sterilization pouches are used for placing instruments in before putting them in the pressure cooker. Always buy bigger sized ones than you think you'll need.

Buy packages that are much bigger than your instruments. 20% of the pouch is sealed on both sides, leaving the room inside smaller than appearing.

Often the most surprising fact for most people, is that if you can sterilize instruments because you have access to an oven, it's more effective to bake them at 450 degrees Fahrenheit for 30 minutes, than it is to soak them in any type of medical or chemical disinfectant.

Let's move on and learn to apply the same techniques to render water drinkable.

MAKING POTABLE WATER

Making drinking water safe can be tricky, but not knowing how is fatal. Boiling is the easiest and most time tested technique. But it doesn't destroy botulism.

When boiling water at low elevation, below 6500 feet, you'll only need boil it for one minute before it's safe. Higher elevations require boiling for a full three minutes.

Boiling can be inconvenient, particularly if you don't have fire, wood, or don't want to give your position away. In instances like these, chlorine and Betadine become the most useful methods.

CHLORINE

The principle agent in most household bleaches, chlorine is easy to use, but it doesn't kill Giardia. This parasite is found in streams and rivers throughout the United States, causing severe diarrhea and abdominal pain.

Regular Clorox bleach, and many of its generic equivalents, come in a standard 5% concentration. Remember to check the label when you're transferring it to a smaller container. Some preparations are much stronger; you don't want to confuse the two. One gallon of bleach will disinfect 3800 gallons of non-cloudy water! (But it only has a 1 year shelf life. The warmer it gets, the faster it goes bad.)

> ### Making Water Drinkable with Chlorine
>
> o   Treat water for 30-45 minutes before drinking.
> o   When using bleach of a 4-6% concentration, add 8 drops per gallon, or 2 drops per liter.
> o   7-10% concentrations require 4 drops per gallon or 1 per liter.
> o   Rarely, only 1% bleach can be found. It requires adding 40 drops per gallon or 10 drops per liter. In this case it is helpful to remember that there are 20 drops in 1ml. For a gallon you will need to add 2ml's, and 0.5ml's for 1 liter.
> o   Write the formula on the Clorox bottle if

BETADINE

One of the best reasons to carry Betadine in your medical bag, is that it can clean wounds and make water drinkable. Two drawbacks are: It takes time to work, and doesn't kill Cryptosporidium, an infection with symptoms similar to Giardia.

Doubling the amount of Betadine, cuts the disinfection time in half. Similarly, if you have difficulty drinking the water because of its taste, you can cut the amount of disinfectant by half, and double the treatment time. I find it easiest to remember that 1ml of Betadine, treats one gallon of water.

Making Water Drinkable with Betadine

- o If the water you are disinfecting is clear, it will require 15 minutes before it's drinkable, 30 minutes if the water is cloudy. *Both of these times must be doubled if the water is colder than 40 degrees Fahrenheit.*
- o Use 16 drops of Betadine per gallon, or 4 drops per liter. You can cut the disinfection time in half by doubling the amount of Betadine you use, but this often makes the water difficult to drink.

Water is so important that you shouldn't take shortcuts, and should always have redundant systems for purification. For highly contaminated water, filter it before you treat it with chlorine or Betadine. Filtration can be as easy as pouring it through a coffee filter, or the kitchen sponge you scavenged earlier. Then run it through two rounds of disinfection: chlorine followed by Betadine.

Now that we've learned how to make even muddy water drinkable; we'll discuss conditions when it's most needed:

HEAT EXHAUSTION & HEAT STROKE

Heat stroke kills 700 people a year - and that's with air-conditioning and modern health care. This is nothing compared to what it's going to be, after those conveniences are decimated.

Heat exhaustion and heat stroke are often thought of separately, but are actually a continuum of the same process. Both occur when the person becomes intolerant to the amount of heat they're exposed to.

Heat stroke refers to a very special condition. The person exhibits specific and disturbing neurological symptoms ranging from confusion to seizures. In both heat stroke and exhaustion, treatment *must* begin in the field.

You've probably thought about how easy it would be to suffer heat exhaustion while bugging out, especially during summer months. Studies done in long distance runners show dehydration alone is enough to cause heat exhaustion. I've seen this occur unexpectedly in Army Rangers returning from a weekend pass. Sometimes the younger ones will have consumed alcohol without having drank enough water, and be unknowingly dehydrated. Then they'll go on a run they usually handle with ease, only to develop heat exhaustion or stroke.

Spray Bottles for Heat Stroke

A THERMOS CAN BE DIFFICULT TO FIND, NOT MANY HOMES HAVE ONE. WHEN YOU'RE IN THE LAUNDRY ROOM AND LOOKING TO PUT BLEACH IN SOMETHING, LOOK FOR A SPRAY BOTTLE. HAIRSPRAY, GLASS CLEANER, ANY WILL WORK. THE BLEACH CAN BE REMOVED LATER AND THE BOTTLE USED AS A SPRAYER OF COLD WATER FOR TREATING HEAT EXHAUSTION.

Humans have two main ways of dissipating heat: radiation and evaporation. Radiation works in the same way a radiator in a car or home does, and can be a two-edged sword. If the environment is hotter than the person, the flow of energy will travel in the wrong direction, and the person will become hotter from their surroundings. Evaporation occurs when the persons heat transfers to the moisture on their skin, and then evaporates away. Humidity is the enemy of both processes.

Normally, 65% of heat is lost from radiation, and 30% from evaporation. As environmental temperature rises, evaporation becomes the predominant mechanism. When it reaches 95 degrees, 95% of heat transfer is from evaporation alone. When the humidity reaches 75%, neither system works, and for all practical purposes heat cannot be dissipated. In this situation people are likely to get heat exhaustion without much physical effort.

Fluids with sugar and electrolytes, along with resting in a cool environment, are often all that are needed for treating heat exhaustion. But when a person starts having neurological symptoms, like visual changes, gait instability, or confusion, the treatment must be aggressive. *Heat stroke has a 30-80% mortality rate.*

Begin by removing the persons clothing and spraying any available liquid on their skin. Fan and place them in a shaded breezy area to promote evaporative cooling. By this time you probably won't have any water left, and may have to fill your spray bottle with urine!!!

If you have ice, chemical cooling packs, or even cold compresses, place them in areas where large blood vessels come near the surface. The neck, arm pits, groin and scalp all work well. This technique avoids shivering, which generates more heat. And decreases the temperature five times faster than a cool environment alone.

Tylenol, aspirin, and ibuprofen *will not work* to lower a persons' temperature in this setting; it's not immune system activation causing the "fever."

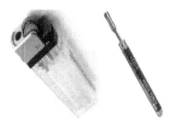 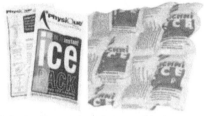

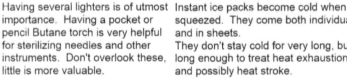

Having several lighters is of utmost importance. Having a pocket or pencil Butane torch is very helpful for sterilizing needles and other instruments. Don't overlook these, little is more valuable.

Instant ice packs become cold when squeezed. They come both individually and in sheets.
They don't stay cold for very long, but long enough to treat heat exhaustion and possibly heat stroke.

In contrast to hypothermia, acclimatization to heat is possible. It typically takes 8-11 days to reach its greatest benefit, and only requires a small amount of exercise. Walking in the heat for two hours a day is often all that's needed for acclimatization to occur.

All of that being said, let's see how cold injures can leave you just as dead:

Dealing with Cold Injuries - Hypothermia & Frostbite

Which would you rather die from: having your brain sizzled, or your blood frozen? The same mechanisms preventing heat exhaustion and stroke (evaporation and radiation,) play equal but opposite roles in cold injuries.

Wet clothes offer a surface for evaporation, and wind accelerates the process. Radiation in this environment is self-explanatory, and staying warm is of prime concern. History is littered with examples of armies too cold to fight. And of soldiers incapacitated by the physical and psychological effects of the freeze.

Children and young adults seem to be resistant to freezing injures. When they do get them, they have fewer disabilities later. Cold injuries can be divided into three major categories: cold/wet, cold/dry, and hypothermia.

Cold / wet Injuries

In general these injuries are dependent on time and temperature. The warmer, the more time required to produce damage.   The colder, the quicker the injury appears.

Chilblain injures can involve the hands and feet, but are most commonly seen on the extremities between a person's joints.   This distribution results from contact with damp clothing over long periods of time.

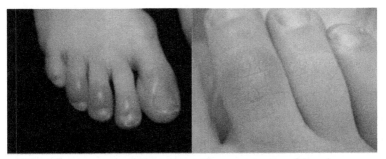

Chilblains are caused by prolonged exposure to cold and humidity. The capillaries beds are damaged, leading to redness, itching, blisters and inflammation.

The area will first turn red, then become swollen, tender and hot to the touch.   Initially the only symptom a person has is excessive itching.   But with repeated exposure the area turns to a reddish-purple, and blisters often begin to form.   With chronic exposure the itching is replaced by a burning pain, one that can last for many years.

Areas enclosing an atmosphere of moderate cold with high humidity are thought to be the cause.   This is why it occurs so often inside rubberized boots and footwear.

Pernio is the name given to the advanced form of chilblain.   Affected areas produce superficial burning and pain.   Sometimes the overlying tissue will slough off, only to leave painful tissue behind. The longer the extremity is exposed to cold, the greater the depth of injury, until eventually trenchfoot develops.

Trenchfoot, also known as immersion foot, generally results from exposures lasting longer than 12 hours, and in water temperatures below 50 degrees. Trenchfoot can even occur in tropical environments, though it takes much longer. Cases like this are mostly seen in shipwreck survivors floating in life rafts.

There are three stages leading to trenchfoot. The first occurs within a few hours or days of the exposure. Here the extremity becomes swollen, numb, discolored and sometimes can be pulseless. The next phase lasts 2-6 weeks, and produces a tingling pain with wide temperature gradients on the effected skin. This is when blistering occurs, and can lead to gangrene. The last stage unfolds over weeks to months. The person may not experience discomfort during this stage. But if exposed to cold again, they get swelling, pain, itching, numbness and loss of skin sensitivity. During this, the skin will usually turn from red to a deep blue and then black.

Trenchfoot usually occurs on land, and immersion foot in water. Both are similar in symptoms and treated the same way. Trenchfoot in particular is worsened with repetitive trauma: walking, standing or sitting for long periods with wet footwear. Both injuries are worsened by malnutrition, depression, and apathy. Trenchfoot usually causes wet gangrene, an injury characterized by infected dead tissue.

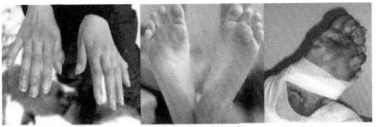

Cold/wet injures can occur on both the hands and feet. Try to leave the blisters intact for as long as possible. They decrease the infection rate by preventing bacteria from entering the underlying tissue.

Trenchfoot is a severe injury. Prohibit exposure to cold while it's healing.

Treatment of trenchfoot begins with carefully drying the feet and warming the body, while at the same time keeping the feet cool. Elevate the feet and put the person on bed rest, fan the area if possible. Try to improve the person's nutritional status by adding vitamin supplementation and a high protein diet. Outside of a hospital setting, it's about all that can be done.

COLD / DRY INJURIES

Tissue damage resulting from the outright freezing of tissue is classified as either frostnip or frostbite.

Frostnip can be thought of as the opposite of sunburn. It occurs when only the superficial layers of the skin are frozen, and doesn't result in later tissue damage or loss. Repeated episodes in the same area often cause dry, scaly, and pealing skin that cracks and becomes sensitive to the cold.   While not a serious injury, repeated episodes can predispose the area to frostbite.

Frostbite occurs when tissue fluids in the skin or underlying tissue get cold enough to freeze and form ice crystals.   Since WW I, frostbite has been the most common cold injury sustained in military operations.

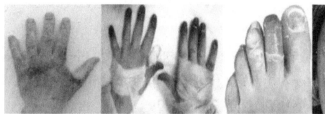

Frostbite ranges in severity and shouldn't be treated with rapid re-warming, unless you can insure it won't be refrozen again. Refreezing vastly increases the tissue damage.

Exposed areas like ear lobes and distal parts of fingers and toes are most vulnerable. Warm clothing prevents this.

At first the affected areas appear as a whitish dry and waxy patches that are insensitive to touch.   Then they become fixed, hard, and non-depressible, especially when over the joints.   Rewarming, regardless of the speed at which it's done, often causes intense pain and swelling with blister formation.

Unlike the treatment of trenchfoot, the treatment of frostbite requires rapid rewarming.   But this must be avoided if there's any chance the extremity will freeze again. Rewarming it, just to have it freeze again, drastically increases the tissue damage.

Trenchfoot is treated with slow rewarming. Frostbite with rapid rewarming. Both treatments can be quite painful.

Rapid rewarming is best accomplished by submerging the extremity in warm water (104-108 degrees) while bringing it through its normal range of motion.

Hypothermia occurs with whole body freezing. The best treatment is avoidance. Solar blankets can be helpful with this and should be standard equipment in your BOB.

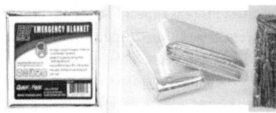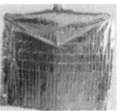

Emergency thermal blankets take up very little room and are inexpensive. The disadvantage is that they can easily give away your position.

Have you ever smelled a rotting wound? Up next: Amputations and Gangrene!

WET & DRY GANGRENE

Gangrene is a potentially life-threatening condition that arises when body tissue dies. It can occur after an injury or infection, but in everyday life is most common in diabetics with poor circulation. It's an important disease for preppers to know about, because cold injuries damage blood vessels, predisposing the person to gangrene.

As more vessels are injured, more dead tissue accumulates. The process can occur slowly, or all at once. In both instances the dead tissue can progress to gangrene.

While there are many types of gangrene, it's easiest to divide them into two forms: wet and dry.

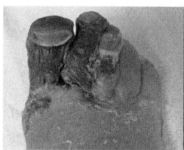 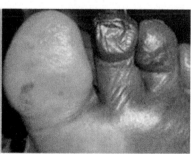

Dry gangrene. Just leave this alone, and cover it. The toes will autoamputate (fall off.)

Wet gangrene. This condition needs antibiotics and possibly amputation. Sepsis may result.

Dry gangrene is the least dangerous. Rarely are infections a significant problem, and the digits will generally fall off on their own.

Wet gangrene includes gas gangrene and necrotizing fasciitis (flesh eating bacteria.) These are serious infections and often lead to sepsis if untreated. Sepsis is a condition where the bacteria from the infection make their way into the bloodstream causing the whole body to react. People used to refer to this as blood poisoning, although I am not quite sure if it's an exact match with sepsis.

Fever and chills are generally the first signs of sepsis. Progression to confusion and shock soon follow. Treatment has to be swift at this stage, antibiotics alone are no longer going to hold off the infection. Amputation is going to be required!

Let's hope this never happens. Let's hope your most serious injuries will be sprains and strains. Those are easiest to treat. And here's how:

SECTION TWO
LUMPS, BUMPS & BROKEN BONES

SPRAINS, STRAINS & AUTOMOBILES

In the field sprains and strains are more common than lacerations or penetrating wounds. Ankle sprains being most common of all. We'll consider these in detail, as the principles of their treatment applies to strains and sprains elsewhere in the body.

Strains are the given name to trauma occurring in tendons, the tissue connecting muscles to bone. Sprains are like strains, but occur in ligaments, the tissue connecting bone to bone. Tendons and ligaments are made of strands of linear connective tissue. Their inelasticity makes them prone to injury when stretched suddenly.

The severity of sprains and strains are categorized by a grading system. It serves as a rough approximation of the degree of damage. It must be remembered that such injuries form a continuum: barely stretched, to completely torn apart.

GRADE ONE

In grade one injuries, the tissue sustains small and often microscopic tears. Even though the spaces between these tears are small, some fill in with blood which eventually clots. This stimulates an inflammatory reaction, turning the clots into new ligament or tendon. Depending upon its severity, the process may take several weeks. Rest, ice, elevation, and an elastic pressure dressings are treatments of choice.

GRADE TWO

Roughly 50% of the fibers have be disrupted, resulting in different degrees of laxity in the joint. Tissue heals through the same inflammatory process described above, but often takes longer, and can be incomplete. Chronic instability, like that seen in a person prone to dislocating their shoulder, may result. Grade two injuries are notorious for causing bruising below the sprain. This can be confusing but is nothing more than the location where the blood has pooled under the force of gravity.

GRADE THREE

Complete disruption of the tissue occurs; the ligament breaks, and the joint becomes unstable. When this happens to tendons, like the Achilles, the muscle is no longer attached to the bone, and the joint cannot be moved in one of its directions. Often third degree sprains and strains require surgery if full function is to return.

For preppers, ankle sprains are of most concern when bugging out. Scattered debris, unstable ground, and unfamiliar terrain can all contribute to twisting the ankle.

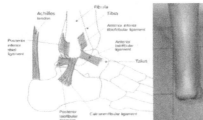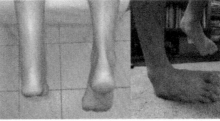

Rupture of the Achilles tendon prevents a person from walking as they can no longer push off with their foot. In the photo in the center you can see where the tendon is no longer attached on the left leg. When the ankle sprains, it usually inverts (right)

GRADE 1 SPRAINS

The ligaments are stretched or slightly torn, causing a mild injury that will improve with light stretching and rest. Some are more severe than others, causing micro-hemorrhaging that results in bruising.   Rest, ice, elevation, and an elastic pressure dressings are treatments of choice.

GRADE 2 SPRAINS

The ligaments are partially torn and fill with blood to different degrees.   Initially these are treated with ice, compression bandages and rest, but often need a splint or cast.

GRADE 3 SPRAINS

Complete disruption of the ligament occurs.   It's sometimes difficult to tell without an X-ray if a bone has been broken.   The joint may fill with blood, particularly the knee, making walking or even weight bearing almost impossible.

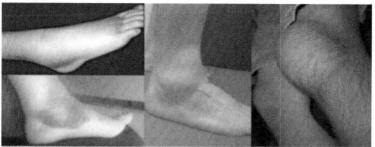

Blood pooling is gravity dependent and tends to collect below the injury. It can't predict severity. Joints fill with fluid causing swelling. When they fill with blood, a serious injury has usually occured. It can be hard to tell if a bone has been broken.

Treatment of grade 1-2 injuries consists of Rest, Ice, Compression wraps, and Elevation. Once referred to by the mnemonic RICE, the treatment is now preceded by a "P," reminding the person to protect the joint from further injury.

For our purposes remember "A PRICE," prompting the addition of anti-inflammatory medication like aspirin or ibuprofen. Remember that Tylenol, known by its generic name as acetaminophen, will treat pain but not inflammation.

If ice is available, apply it for 20 minutes at a time. Four to eight treatments in the first 24 hours work best. Be sure to put a thin piece of fabric between the ice and skin to prevent cold burns.

Ice is unlikely to be accessible though. In this case you'll want to use tight, but not constrictive, heavily reinforced elastic wraps. After 24 hours, switch from ice or tight wraps to heat treatments. During this phase of the trauma, you're no longer trying to stop swelling, but trying to increase the necessary blood perfusion required for healing.

Use ice in the first 24 hours, heat thereafter. For added pain relief in any condition, you can give Tylenol along with ibuprofen or aspirin, but never aspirin or ibuprofen together. This will cause stomach upset and sometimes bleeding.

Joint protection is best accomplished with bracing. Air splints are excellent for this. They can be used for all grades of sprains and strains, as well as for the initial treatment of broken bones.

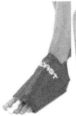 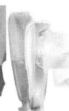 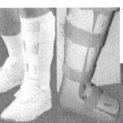 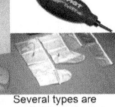

Aircast's for feet are often mistaken for those used in ankle sprains.	A single aircast is all that is needed. They are used for support and protection from further injury. They have the advantage of fitting over shoes & boots.	A "fracture walker" is best, but it takes up too much room in your kit.	Several types are available and some come with an insufflation bulb. Can be used to treat some fractures w/o casting.

The truth of the matter is, if you injure a lower extremity while bugging out, you aren't going to make it far. You'll have to "borrow" an automobile.   Likely there won't be one around.   So when you plan the trip to your BOL, factor in safe rest areas where you can shelter until you're back on your feet.

Bugging out time is like the dark night of the soul for a zombie prepper.   It's the time when the gravity of what's happened hasn't totally hit you, but your senses are still glazed over.   Choose every step carefully, pay attention to everything in your environment.   Here is what to do if your back, knees or feet are killing you:

BACK, KNEE, & FOOT PAIN

We think it was probably the lack of rubber during times of war that did it. We can't be sure, but the high prevalence of knee and foot pain experienced by WWII survivors may have been from inadequate or unavailable foot wear. Some things just can't be replaced in an apocalypse. During WWII it was shoes and eye glasses. For us it will be shoes, glasses, contacts, and our daily medications – *among others of course.*

You likely already know a great deal about footwear. We'd like to add to that knowledge by showing you how to tweak your shoes and boots to compensate for heavy packs and long distance treks. We'd like to teach you effective ways of dealing with runners toe and sprained ankles, so you'll have complete mobility and be able to bug out to any place at any time.

HOW TO ADJUST YOUR FOOT ARCHES TO ELIMINATE BACK, KNEE AND FOOT PAIN

Sometimes you have to move. Sometimes there's just no choice. But this isn't possible with throbbing feet and aching knees. On the run from the decomposing hordes, you'll want to know how to treat these conditions.

Because statistically speaking, they're going to happen to at least one person in your group.

The good news is it's easy!   The bad news is that if a prepper doesn't know how to do this, then their knee pain may never resolve - no matter what they do.

Knee pain often begins in the feet, so abnormalities there must be corrected first.   We all are born with a bony arch in our foot, one that normally acts as a shock absorber. During midstride we balance directly over one foot while our other swings forward.   Typically, the arch collapses a little under our weight.   This "bounciness" prevents the knee from rotating inward or outward and torqueing on the ligaments holding it together.   It's not difficult to imagine then, that if the arch of a foot either collapses too much or too little, those torsional forces will be transferred to the knee with every step.

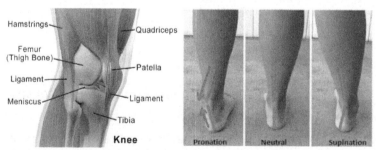

Knee pain often begins with unrecognized problems in the feet. Preppers need to know how to treat these conditions, otherwise their pain is unlikely to improve. The first step is to determine if your foot is rolling too far inward or outward when you walk. The second is to fix your footwear to compensate for the unwanted motion. Doing this is quick & easy!

If your arch collapses too easily, or if your foot is already flat, then your foot will abnormally roll inward. This condition is called over-pronation.   And when it occurs the knee must rotate in the opposite direction to compensate - otherwise your leg would not remain straight. But you take thousands of steps every day. And if each one of them is torqueing on the ligaments and tendons of your knee, it won't be long before pain sets in.

As you're reading this, take off one of your shoes and look at the sole. If the inside edge is worn down more than the outside edge - you over-pronate!

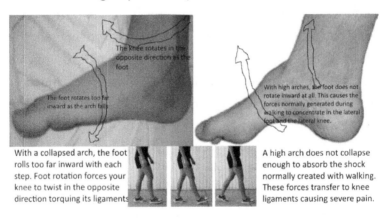

The knee rotates in the opposite direction as the foot

The foot rotates too far inward as the arch fails

With high arches, the foot does not rotate inward at all. This causes the forces normally generated during walking to concentrate in the lateral foot and the lateral knee.

With a collapsed arch, the foot rolls too far inward with each step. Foot rotation forces your knee to twist in the opposite direction torquing its ligaments

A high arch does not collapse enough to absorb the shock normally created with walking. These forces transfer to knee ligaments causing severe pain.

Likewise, if your arch is too high and doesn't collapse when you walk, excessive forces will be transferred to the outside portion of your foot and knee resulting in pain. Look at your sole again. Is the outside edge more heavily worn than the inside edge? If it is, then your foot isn't absorbing the shock it should be.

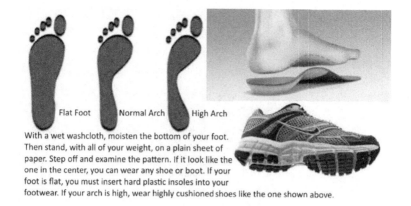

Flat Foot   Normal Arch   High Arch

With a wet washcloth, moisten the bottom of your foot. Then stand, with all of your weight, on a plain sheet of paper. Step off and examine the pattern. If it look like the one in the center, you can wear any shoe or boot. If your foot is flat, you must insert hard plastic insoles into your footwear. If your arch is high, wear highly cushioned shoes like the one shown above.

To see if a person suffering from knee pain has either of these conditions, or to see if their foot is normal, perform the "wet test" described above. If the person's foot turns out to be flat, you can easily fix it by inserting hard plastic arch supports into their shoes.

If their arch doesn't collapse at all, then they need very spongy shoes to absorb the shock of walking. Choosing or modifying the best footwear for painful feet and knees is that simple. It takes only a few minutes, and can make all the difference between whether or not a person makes it to their bug-out-location.

PREVENTING & TREATING BACK, KNEE, AND FOOT PAIN CAUSED BY BACKPACKS

It's true people aren't getting back pain from their packs like they used to. Improved designs have seen to that. But they are getting more and more hip, knee and foot pain. The good news is that you can treat these

195

conditions quickly, helping to ensure you and your group make it all the way to your bug-out-location in a timely manner.

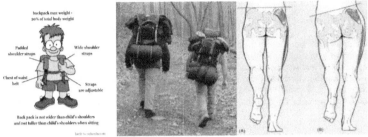

Back pain caused by a heavy backpack is still a problem for children, but is becoming rare in adults. Improvements in design allow more weight to be carried comfortably. But this is resulting in an increase of hip, knee, and foot pain. The extra weight pulls on the lateral leg muscles, twists the knees, and flattens the feet - which roll inward.

If you're a runner, iliotibial band syndrome is probably familiar to you.   But it's common in preppers also. With every step, carrying even a little extra weight can put stress on your lateral leg muscles.   And since these muscles insert around the outside of your knee, the force pushing down from the weight can easily transfer to there and case pain.

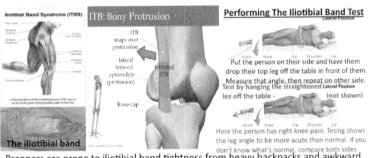

Preppers are prone to iliotibial band tightness from heavy backpacks and awkward fitting bug-out-bags. Perform the band test to see if this is the cause of your knee or hip pain. If the angle is less on the painful side, a tight band is likely the problem.

Placing a pillow between your knees when you sleep can help treat this problem.   However, the prepper must also correct for any foot problems, or the condition will never resolve.   You'll want to check to see if the extra weight is also causing your foot arch to collapse.

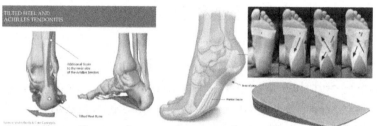

Bug-out-bags and heavy packs commonly cause two foot problems - plantar fasciitis & Achilles tendonitis. The extra weight can cause the foot arch to collapse and roll inward (overpronation). Low-Dye taping (upper right) can relieve a preppers pain from plantar fasciitis, and a thin heel lift can improve Achilles tendonitis - until they get to their BOL. For both conditions, a permanent solution is hard plastic orthotics.

If you use a heel lift to take the pressure off your Achilles tendon, start with a thin one.   Just a little lift can be a big shock to the body.   But it can also help you get to where you're going, so you can formally address the problem with hard plastic orthotics later.

RUNNERS TOE

Have you ever had someone show up for a trek through a dense wet forest or jungle with a brand new pair of combat boots?   It almost never goes well.

It's a different story for preppers who are sporting boots they've broken in for years.   Footwear that fits like a glove, and they drag with them everywhere.   Point being, those aren't the people I'm talking about.   Newbies and brand new boots always slow everyone down.   As they begin stepping on the large rounded logs decorating the forest floor, their feet slip slightly within their boots.   That torqueing action translates directly to the skin of their soles and toe pads.   Add a little water or damp socks to the mix, and blisters can't help but to form.

New footwear also presents a second problem – runners toe.

A subungual hematoma, or runner's toe, is a common condition seen in runners, skiers, hikers, and military personnel.   It's caused by downward pressure on the nail, often from tight fitting footwear.   Preppers are likely to see this condition in people they travel with.   It's a frequent ailment in those not used to hiking.

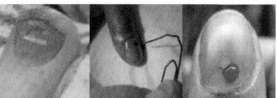

| Often caused by tight fitting boots or shoes. The pain produced is much greater than what you might first expect. | It's the result of just a little bit of blood collecting under the nail of a toe or a finger. The pressure must be released. | Heat up a paper clip with a lighter and press it against the nail for 1-2 seconds. Keep doing this until a hole is made. | Leaving the hot metal on the nail for more than a second causes pain. Only a little blood will come out, but the pain relief is immediate. |

I'd see this condition frequently in skiers with thigh fitting boots. There's no give in those. The force of even a small bump transmits immediately to the nail of the big toe. Before long, blood begins to collect in the nail bed. Decompressing the trapped blood is easy and will result in immediate pain relief.

Runners toe can also occur on the fingers after a crush injury. Pooling of blood underneath the nail plate causes its separation from the bed, and is nearly always painful. In both cases, the pressure can be relieved by burning a hole in the nail with a heated paperclip. The trick is to leave the hot wire on the nail only for a second or two at a time.

Longer than that and the heat will dissipate across the nail's surface and cause pain. Repeatedly applying the paperclip in short intervals to the hole you've created, will eventually cause it to penetrate completely through. Only a small amount of blood will be released, but if done within

36-48 hours of the injury, the pain relief will be immediate. Any longer than that, and the blood will have already clotted, in which case you just let it resolve on its own. Puncturing a hole at that point will do little.

If you don't have a paperclip, you can use the safety pin that comes with your triangular bandage, or better yet, a cautery pen.

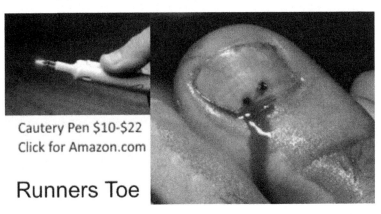

Cautery Pen $10-$22
Click for Amazon.com

Runners Toe

Battery powered devices, these cautery pens are inexpensive at $10-15 and handy to have in your medical kit. The cheapest places to find them are fishing and sporting goods stores. Where apparently they're used for fly tying and other hobbies.

You can be a hero with this trick! So you might want to try bartering with the person before performing it. Because with the next ailment... no one is going to walk away a winner.

BREAKING BONES BAD

Soft tissue injuries can involve the skin, muscle, ligaments, and tendons; but spare the bone they surround. Sprains, strain, muscle tears and bruises all fall within this category.

The difficulty is trying to decide if the trauma has resulted in a grade 2 or 3 sprain, or if the underlying bone has been broken. Swelling along long bones, like those of the upper and lower arms, can be challenging. Without X-rays or an obvious deformity, separating out bruised tissue from broken bones can be a problem for anyone in health care.

The rule in the field, the one specific for preppers, is to treat the injury like a fracture if you're unsure. You really can't go wrong with this approach.

Telling the difference between a broken bone and an injury limited to the soft tissues can be difficult. When in doubt, treat an injury as if it's fractured.

Signs that would tip you toward thinking "broken bone" are excessive swelling accompanied by obvious deformity. Loss of power, discoloration, excessive pain, inability to move the injured part, or feeling the abnormal outline of the bone are also clues. When the patient hears the bone snap at the time of trauma, or can feel the ends of the bone grating together, the diagnosis is obvious.

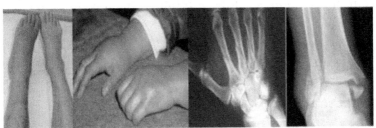

Comparing one limb with the other will often reveal a deformity and points to an obvious fracture (left.) Other times it can be difficult, especially in areas like the hand that tend to swell.

The X-ray of the hand above might correspond to the injury to its left, but without the film it's difficult to tell. In the field it's best to treat the injury as a fracture. Same applies to the ankle.

FRACTURE TYPES

Fractures come in 4 basic varieties: simple or closed, compound or open, complicated and greenstick.

SIMPLE FRACTURES, CLAVICLE AND RIB FRACTURES

If the skin is intact, the fracture's closed.   Simple or closed fractures are those which the surface of the skin hasn't been slit open by broken bone.   Closed injuries are most common.   The swelling and deformity can range from hardly noticeable, to completely obvious.

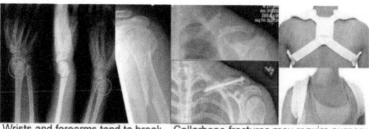

Wrists and forearms tend to break easily. Treat injuries with excessive tenderness or swelling as if broken (left). Bones can break into sharp shards (right) & pierce the skin.

Collarbone fractures may require surgery if really displaced (top left) but this won't be possible in the field. Instead use a figure 8 brace, or make one from a bed sheet, to pull the shoulders back & out.

Collarbone fractures require special attention. They can't be casted.   Immobilization is the best that can be done.   95% heal on their own and don't require surgery. Some are so fragmented or displaced, like the one shown above in the middle, that surgical pinning is required.   Most clavicle breaks heal quickly and may be aided by placing the person in a figure-of-eight brace, shown above on the far right.

It was once thought that this type of bracing helped displaced fractures heal by pulling the shoulders back, so the ends of the bone could re-approximate.   Then studies showed identical healing rates in those treated with a simple sling; and the figure-of-eight fell out of favor.   Many of us still use it though; the pain control seems to be better compared to a conventional sling.

If you are without any supplies, you can sometimes use a bed sheet.   While it is best to use a 4-6 inch elastic bandage in place of a figure-of-eight brace, in a pinch you can use bed sheet strips, or an entire sheet as one whole bulky dressing.   Always anchor the strip or elastic bandage to the arm opposite the injury.

Begin by wrapping the good upper arm a few times before making an "8" with the dressing around the person. Have the patient put his hands on his hips to help get the desired tension.   Remember that if you are using non-elastic bed sheets, the anchoring wrap around the good arm must be a little loose to prevent constriction and subsequent swelling.

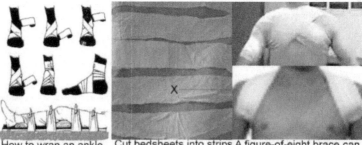

How to wrap an ankle with an elastic bandage (top) - Without supplies stabilize leg with towels

Cut bedsheets into strips if you don't have dressings. Cut one end to the X, then use flaps to tie it.

A figure-of-eight brace can be made with 4-6 inch Ace bandage. Start it by anchoring it on the good arm.

The figure-of-eight can cause its own discomfort and is often cumbersome to adjust. Even after completely healed, most clavicle fractures will produce a noticeable bump under the skin in the area where the bone was broken, regardless of the type of sling used.

Whichever you decide on, continue immobilization for one to two weeks, or until the majority of the pain is gone. Range-of-motion exercises, with pendulum arm rotation, can be started as soon as pain allows. Progression to active range-of-motion and strengthening exercises should continue over the next four to eight weeks.

RIB FRACTURES

The crushing sensation of broken ribs can be tearfully painful and immobilizing. They're frequently caused by falls, and remind you of their presence with every cautious breath. Tight elastic bandages or rib belts can help contain the pain, but also increase the risk of developing pneumonia.

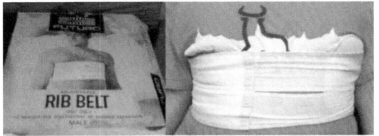

The treatment of rib fractures with rib belts fell out of favor in medicine for many years. People were taking shallow breaths and developing pneumonia. Remember to take several deep breaths an hour. Rib belts can aid with pain control and mobility.

When a rib is broken, the natural tendency is to breathe shallowly, and rib belts encourage this. But we normally inhale germs throughout the day, and need to clear them periodically from our lungs. We do this by breathing deeply and coughing from time to time, but don't take notice. This reflex is inhibited when we're in pain and when wearing a rib belt. If you can remind yourself to breathe deeply a couple of times an hour while the belt is on, an infection is less likely to occur.

<u>Side Note</u>:   Consequences of Contusions & Broken Ribs

World War II survivors can teach zombie preppers a lot about injuries occurring in bizarre and difficult times. They seemed magnetic at times. Attracting everything from free falling objects and ricocheting shrapnel, to earth-rolling blast waves. In the wake they'd always find chest trauma, a condition that has never been a stranger to war.

Lung Contusions & Fluid in the Lung Sacs (Alveoli)

Found in conditions ranging from lung contusions to altitude illness, fluid buildup within the lung sacs where air exchange takes place (alveoli) can occur for a variety of reasons.   Chest trauma not being the least of them.

Contusions or bruises of the lung are usually a consequence of some type of blunt force trauma.   A hematoma or blood collection forms deep within the pulmonary tissue.   Ribs protect the lungs to some degree, but in living creatures they have an inherent give or elasticity.

This rebound capacity causes the force behind the impact to be taken up by the lungs.   As the ribs smack up against the delicate tissue, the force transfers, and the ribs quickly recoil back to normal position.   But sometimes this slapping effect exceeds its limit, and the ribs simply break.

The sharp shards of bone left behind slice through the lung, and air begins leaking out.   A pneumothorax builds, and the lung collapses.   There's no requirement that ribs must be fractured for lung bruising to occur.

Broken and bruised ribs are equally painful.   But bruised ribs don't fragment into sharp shards, so generally they don't cause air leaks.

If bruising of the lung has occurred, you'll want to expect that the person may cough up blood in a few days.

Remember this always looks worse than it is. The blood is coming from bleeding that occurred at time of the accident and has since stopped. Coughing is just a way the collection expels itself. All you'll need to do is check for pneumothorax (the specifics on how to do this is coming up.) Not finding one, you simply reassure the patient and let them know they are going to be sore for a while.

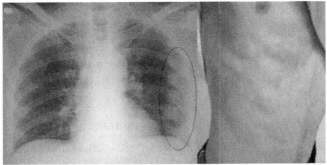

Rib fractures are very painful, because everytime you breathe, the broken bone moves up and down. People then take small breaths to limit the pain.

Fortunately, the majority of rib injuries don't result in pneumothorax. Instead, the main danger comes from the pain they cause. It discourages the person from breathing deeply. With the lung not completely filling with air from time to time, the person is predisposed to getting pneumonia.

Take Home Message:

1. When a rib is broken, the natural tendency is to breathe shallowly to avoid the sharp stabbing pain inherent with this type of fracture.

2. This is a problem, because we normally inhale germs throughout the day, and need to clear them periodically from our lungs. We do this by breathing deeply and coughing from time to time. But this reflex is suppressed when we're in pain, and when we're wearing a rib belt.

3. If you can remind your patient to breathe deeply a couple of times an hour, and are sure they will do this while the belt is on, then an infection is less likely to occur - and it might be safe for them to use one of these pain relieving devices.

BROKEN RIBS TO BROKEN FINGERS & LONG BONES

Broken fingers and toes are also incredibly painful. Both have a tendency to move around more than long bones, creating pain each time.

Bone setting techniques are as aged as society. The Japanese were particularly good at it. When one Ju-Jitsu school would brawl with another, bones were sure to be broken.   The following day the winning school would set the fractures of their adversaries.

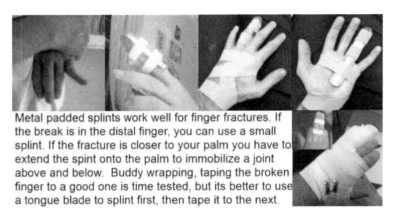

Metal padded splints work well for finger fractures. If the break is in the distal finger, you can use a small splint. If the fracture is closer to your palm you have to extend the spint onto the palm to immobilize a joint above and below. Buddy wrapping, taping the broken finger to a good one is time tested, but its better to use a tongue blade to splint first, then tape it to the next.

For those interested in all things martial, know that a collarbone fracture is especially painful.   Many schools of martial arts have techniques for breaking them.   The opponent will quickly drop to the ground in pain, and their shoulder will become useless.   I have some personal experience with this... it's effective.   (I've never tried it on a zombie though.)

Like all medical advice given in this book, it should only be followed when conventional medical care will not be available. Don't realign a bone for instance, if medical care will be available. That being said, if you do have to set a bone, you might want to use a hematoma block.

NON-UNION

When a bone has been broken, and its ends are still touching, it has a good chance of healing with a cast.   If the broken ends are not aligned, or are not touching properly, the bone may not heal.   This condition is called "non-union."

Some fractures may never heal if not reset to their proper positions.   Bone setting   is known as "reduction" in the medical world.   Open reduction is something a surgeon does through an operation.   A pin or metal fixation device is inserted, bringing the ends together, and fixing the bone in place.

In the field, only closed reduction is possible.   Here the bones are moved around by hand and worked back into correct alignment before the cast is applied.   Doing this can

211

be painful and challenging. It probably shouldn't be entertained unless the broken bone has cut off the blood supply to the rest of the extremity.

Some fractures will cause this, they'll pinch or crowd off the blood supply distal to the break. Realigning the bone by moving the broken ends close to one another, should be attempted whenever this occurs.

Most people know how to feel for a radial pulse, if it's present after a break, you're probably okay. If not, try to set the bone with the intention of restoring the pulse.

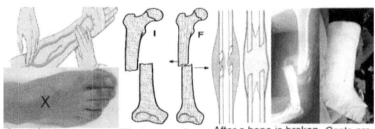

Some fractures can damage or pinch off blood vessels, so check for them distal to the break. X marks 1 pulse

The bone ends should be touching for bone healing to occur, at times you need to set them.

After a bone is broken a callus forms, and the bone heals (left). If the ends are not touching, the bone may not heal (right).

Casts are often needed for bones to heal.

HEMATOMA BLOCK

This is a technique used to allow painless manipulation of broken bones and avoid the need for hospital anesthesia. It's normally only appropriate for fractures of the distal arms and distal legs.

Most broken bones don't become displaced.   When they do, the space separating the fragments fills with blood. Having been released by the damaged blood vessels within the bone, the blood collects into a ball shaped hematoma.

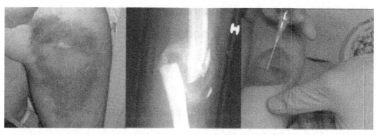

Hematomas in soft tissues are bruises (left.) They also form around the broken ends of a bone (center.) To block the nerve endings so the bone can be set, clean the skin and advance the needle until it hits bone, then inject 10 ml lidocaine (right.)

Injection of lidocaine through the skin and into the hematoma produces pain relief.   This allows the bone to be painlessly manipulated back into place.   Avoid doing this with fractures of the collarbone, because you can accidently hit the underlying lung and collapse it.

Under sterile conditions you can insert a needle attached to a syringe of lidocaine, and advance it until it makes contact with the bone.   Aim for where you think the bone separation is, and then inject the lidocaine.   Wait longer than usual for the medicine to take effect, and inject more than usual.   It takes a while to start working, but may relieve the pain enough that you can work the bone back into some type of acceptable alignment.

GREENSTICK A.K.A CHALKSTICK FRACTURES

Greenstick fractures occur mostly in children and young adolescents. Their bones aren't as brittle as adult's, and the bone's covering is thicker. The ends remain attached with this fracture, but are often offset at an angle.

The bone covering, called periosteum, contains nerve endings and is responsible for the pain caused in fractures. Normally a physician will grasp both ends of the broken bone, and with a twist of the wrists, break the periosteal attachment so the bone doesn't heal at an angle. This can be quite difficult to do without an X-ray and analgesia. It's unlikely you would ever have to set a greenstick fracture, usually you'll need an X-ray to know this type of break is present in the first place.

Regardless of the fracture type, if you don't feel comfortable setting it, then just cast the extremity when the swelling goes down (use a splint until then.) It may heal at an angle, but at least it will heal. Recent studies have shown that greenstick fractures that are not re-broken, may heal better in a removable splint than a cast. Take a few minutes and watch some YouTube videos on splinting, and casting with plaster.

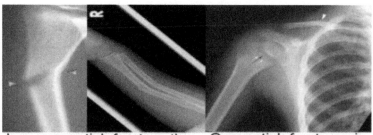

In a greenstick fracture the bone is held together by its covering. If not rebroken, the bone will heal at an angle.

Greenstick fractures in children are common & don't need rebreaking if in the collarbone.

MORE ON CASTING AND SPLINTING

Casting is tricky in the field. You probably won't have the plaster or fiberglass needed. Pre-manufactured air casts are available, and take up little room. They work best if the patient can remain immobile. Before Appling any constrictive casting, swelling in the extremity must be allowed to resolve, otherwise the cast will fit too loosely later.

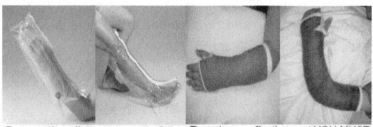

Pneumatic splints are easy to fit in a kit. They don't provide the stability needed to be used as a traditional cast, but may be all that you have. Try reinforcing it with boards & tape

To make an effective cast YOU MUST CAST THE JOINT ABOVE & BELOW THE BREAK! The cast on the left will not work for a forearm fracture, the elbow & wrist must be immobilized, as they are above and below the break.

Magazines, even thick rolls of newspaper, can be used as a splint or makeshift cast. Reinforced with duct tape, they can be left on for the duration. In a psychiatric ward where I once worked, we had to cast (actually splint) patients with newspapers and tape, because they would often assault one another with their "fiber-glassed" arms. This worked well until a patient took off the newspaper and honed it into a cone, then stabbed a person in the abdomen with it. None of us saw that coming. But it's something to keep in mind if you're treating a person that's a threat to themselves or someone else.

If someone in your group has had a cast before, enlist their help in the process. They will know how it should fit and feel, having worn one for two months themselves.

If you do decide to buy casting material, purchase the old fashion plaster type. The fiberglass variety is difficult to remove, dries up in the package quickly, and is nearly impossible to remove without a special saw. Plaster casting comes apart when it gets wet, so it must be covered with plastic while bathing. But this can also work to your advantage. When the time comes to remove it, soak it instead of trying to saw it off.

When Is The Fracture Healed?

Upper Limb	Lower Limb	
6-8 weeks	12-16 weeks	**Adult**
3-4 weeks	6-8 weeks	**Child**

Children are in a constant and dynamic state of growth. Their fractures heal quickly, about twice the rate of an older adolescent or adult. For fractures of the arm, their casts should be removed after three or four weeks, while the adolescent and adult will require six to eight weeks before healing is complete.

OPEN FRACTURES

Compound or open fractures occur when a sharp bone fragment has pierced through the skin. Fortunately these don't occur often, as they usually require a tremendous amount of force. Often the real problem is in trying to figure out if the skin above the fracture has been broken by a sharp bone fragment, or by the trauma that caused the break.

Without an X-ray it can be difficult. This is important because the natural impulse is to probe the wound to find out. Doing this is of little value. And almost guarantees the patient will get a deep infection of the bone. So keep the wound sterile, especially for the first 24-48 hours while it's sealing over.

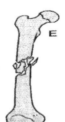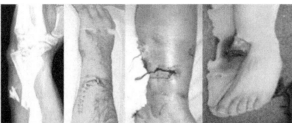

Sometimes bone will break producing sharp fragments. Even with surgical correction there are high infection rates. Without surgical care, these wounds are grave. The best you can do is cover it with a sterile dressing and try to reduce it when muscle spams have resolved. ONLY do this if medical care will never be possible.

My recommendation would be to splint, not cast an open fracture, and to keep the extremity immobilized. If you put a cast over it, you won't be able to see if the wound has become infected. The person can become septic and die before you even know what's happening. In this case, a person can really die from a broken bone.

Let's move on to the creepy crawlies of the world. Spiders, snakes and attorneys:

SECTION THREE
POISON PLANTS, CRITTERS, & BUGS FROM HELL

INSECTS & ARACHNIDS

MOSQUITOS

Even if you're used to it, traveling over land in the summer can be brutal, especially in the Southern United Sates. It's not just the heat, it's the mosquitos. And while they don't carry malaria, they deposit a protein under your skin that will make you itch like a crack addict.

Heat a spoon and hold it to an insect bite to relieve the itching.

Ticks, leeches, and mosquitos all inject an anesthetic into your skin when they attach. This allows them to go unnoticed until they are done feeding.

It's easiest to wear repellant, but it's not something you'd think about during a tsunami or reactor meltdown. There is a quick trick that can help with itchy mosquito bites. Take a spoon and warm it over a flame. Press the hot spoon against the bite and hold it down for a few seconds. Don't heat the spoon so much that it burns your skin, but get it hot. The heat will denature and destroy the itchy protein the mosquito has left behind.

Packing a mosquito net is a no loose endeavor. If it isn't needed, it can always be used to catch fish!

If you live in the South pack a mosquito net in your bug-out-bag. A few years back, in effort to control malaria in underdeveloped countries, the World Health Organization tried widespread distribution of nets to indigenous populations. It didn't work. The nets were inevitably used for fishing.

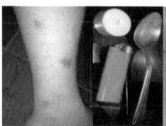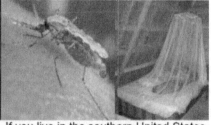

Heat the spoon until hot but not burning. Press it against the bite for a few seconds to a minute. The itching will stop in a minute or two.

If you live in the southern United States, pack a mosquito net in your BOB. In other locations in the U.S., it may not be necessary for insects, BUT WORKS GREAT AS A FISHING NET!

TICKS

Best known for spreading Rocky Mountain Spotted Fever and Lyme disease, ticks are a common problem. For some reason when they lodge in the back of the neck, they

221

can cause a type of ascending paralysis, though do so rarely. This is when a person's feet start to become numb, and the numbness gradually climbs upward toward the head. Removal of the tick will resolve these unusual symptoms.

Trying to remove ticks has gone through a long and troubled evolution in America. While it's agreed that removing the entire tick, and not leaving any of the head or mouth in the wound is a priority, few of us have been able to do this most times.

Squeezing the tick's body will cause it to regurgitate stomach contents into the person, often with disease causing microbes in the mix. So if you do choose to use tweezers, grab the head as close to the skin possible. But don't use tweezers if you can avoid it.

Smothering the tick by covering it with Vaseline has also been tried, but usually results in regurgitation before self-extraction. Getting it to back out by holding a hot match to its rear might work at times, but most often only burns the patient. Many of us feel it's best to inject lidocaine under the tick using a small bore insulin style syringe/needle, then pull it out.

This technique has several advantages. The wheel of lidocaine under the skin produces an upward pressure that prevents stomach contents from entering, even when its body is accidently squeezed. Moreover, if the tick does not back out on its own, and has to be pulled out with tweezers, the remaining parts can be cut out with a scalpel because the area will be deadened.

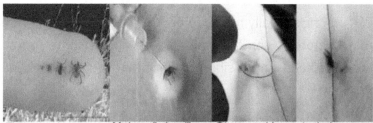

Ticks can be so small, they're almost impossible to see, especially in hairy areas.	Make a "wheel" with lidocaine and wait for the tick to back out. Cut the head out if needed.	Straw and lasso technique. Pin the tick inside a cut straw, and tie a thread around it. Pull the tick out with the lasso, it won't regurgitate this way.

If you don't have lidocaine, you can have someone hold a straw ever the critter and encircle it with sewing thread.   Gently tighten a knot around the straw as it's slowly retracted.   You will be left with a lassoed tick.   The knot will prevent stomach regurgitation, and you can use the thread to pull the little guy out.

Ticks can carry a variety of diseases, most of which produce rashes, and respond well to doxycycline taken for 14 days.   If a person has a rash that involves the palms, and that was not preceded by a common head cold, a tick borne illness may be the cause.   Give the person an antibiotic. Doxycycline works best, and the infection usually resolves.

All in all, doxycycline is probably the most versatile drug for use in the wilderness.   If you can only pack one antibiotic make it doxycycline.   It predisposes people to sunburn and has some restrictions with pregnancy, but is easy to come by and works for many ailments.   If nowhere else, you can find it in a pet store.   More about antibiotics in the upcoming "Fish-i-cillin" chapter.

A tick usually needs to be attached to you for 24-36 hours before it can transmit disease. But some are so small, it's nearly impossible to notice that you've even been bit.

Tularemia is another common wilderness ailment. It can be transmitted by ticks, rabbits, and wild hogs. It's incredibly infectious, and results in a person's lymph nodes swelling up so much, that they look like abscesses.

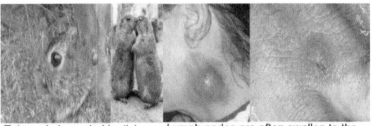

Tularemia is carried by ticks who have fed on infected rabbits or rodents, or by the animals themselves. Don't eat slow moving rabbits, they're ill!

Lymph nodes are often swollen to the point they look like abscesses. Doxycycline treats most tick borne diseases including Lyme disease. Also used for Anthrax, Pneumonia & Malaria.

Doxycycline works well for this too. In bunnies and hogs the disease is usually contracted when skinning and cleaning the animal. Both tend to be an outdoor food source, so care must be taken during the preparation to protect yourself.

LICE

Head and body lice look alike; both need to feed on your blood to survive. They prefer living near the heat of the host, and will die at room temperature if they fall off.

Particularly problematic is the itching they cause. Scratching leads to minor abrasions in the skin, which allows the entry of bacteria and later infection.

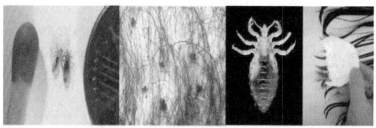

Head and body lice look alike, although body lice have adapted to attach themselves to clothing. Lice must feed on blood to survive. If they become seperated from the host, they die at room temperature. Infestations are common when people are packed closely together. If medicated shampoos aren't availible, you'll need to shave your head!

Unexplained itching should prompt a search for lice nits (eggs.) They can be seen in the seams of an infected person's clothing or scalp. Once attached, nits take a week or two to hatch. It's important to remember this, because simply washing your clothes will not destroy the eggs.

You must place your clothing, sleeping bag, cushions and all other fabrics into a completely airtight plastic bag for two full weeks. Without medicated shampoo's to remove the lice and nits, the only way to get them out of your hair and scalp is to shave your head. Often your body hair and eyebrows will need to be included.

I highly recommend keeping Lindane, known by its trade name Kwell, in your medical kit or BOB. It works for head, body, and pubic lice. It also treats scabies.

SCABIES AND FLEAS

Scabies are very small little critters that cause quite a bit of itching, particularly in the hands. The female burrows into the top layer of skin, the epidermis, and lays 10 to 20 eggs before dying. Larvae emerge from the tunnels three weeks later. Then the females are impregnated and burrow again, repeating the cycle.

Itching is severe and worse at night. The burrows resemble black threads that end in very small blisters called vesicles. They occur on the fingers and wrists, and are most noticeable in the skin webbing between fingers. Treatment with Lindane is most effective.

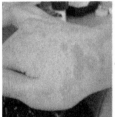 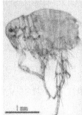 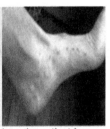

Scabies cause intense itching, especially at night. They often leave burrows in the webbing between the fingers that look like little black threads. The wrists can be involved.

Fleas are blood-suckers that have spread diseases like plague and typhus in the past. Their bites can look like hives, and are very itchy. Treat the itching with Benadryl.

Fleas are also blood sucking pests. They've spread horrific disease throughout history, causing untold human suffering. Their bites are often mistaken for hives, as they look very similar and intensely itch. Fleas typically attack humans only when there are no pets around for them to feed on.

They don't tend to stick to humans. With the exception of the scalp, we don't have enough body hair to hold them. Instead they jump up to our feet or ankles, feed, and disappear. They leave red and itchy raised sores that look very similar to the hives one sees with allergic reactions.

For some reason garlic repels fleas. You can apply some to your lower legs, or to your pet to prevent bites. Then try to revoke their birth certificates by making a flea trap.

I highly recommend including a topical steroid cream like cortisone for your kit. It can be used for almost all skin conditions, except infections.

Fleas are attracted to heat. So start the construction of your trap by placing a candle next to you, your pet, or your furniture if you are sure you can leave it unattended. The flame will fry them. But this can be a fire hazard, and has obvious limitations. For this reason I suggest constructing the bowl/soap/water trap instead.

Find something that can hold water like a pan or bucket. First add water and then soap. You'll know you've added enough when the color of the water starts to change. Slide the bowl under a heat source. A lamp works well. The fleas will be attracted to the warmth, and eventually fall into the solution. The soap makes them sink. Use lots of soap if you have it.

If you don't have a lamp, put the soapy water in a couple of cups, and set them on a windowsill. The heat of the sun will work as your heat source.

Benadryl and topical cortisone creams can be used to treat the bites. Calamine, aloe, and even homemade citrus sprays have found effective. Watch carefully for infections. They can be caused either by the bite, or the scratching they trigger.

CHIGGERS

Also called red bugs, berry bugs, and harvest mites, chiggers are a type of mite related to ticks. They are most numerous in early summer when weeds and grass are most thick and abundant.

Their larva attach to various animals including humans. They feed on the top layer of skin and cause intense itching. Generally found in the Southern United States, they're nearly microscopic, measuring 0.4 mm, and are colored with a chrome-orange hue.

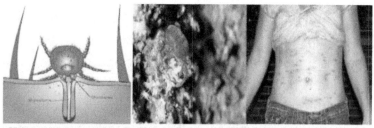

Chigger bites usually occur on belt lines, ankles, or the webbing spaces between fingers. They pierce the skin and release a digestive enzyme that liquifies epidermal cells. The "bite" starts off as a red bump that progresses to a purplish sore, often surrounded by a clear blister. These can last for weeks, and produce intense itching.

After crawling onto a person's skin, they inject digestive enzymes that break down skin cells. They don't actually "bite," but rather form a hole and chew up tiny parts of the inner skin. Severe irritation and swelling soon follow. The treatment is the same as for fleas, though chigger sores last much longer.

ANTS, BEES AND WASPS

This delightful group of insects all belong to the hymenoptera family. This is important, because if a person is allergic to one of the family, they're allergic to all.

All three can sting, including ants. Ants bite too… but only so they can hold onto the animal while stinging. Wasps seem to be more allergenic than bees, but all three may cause allergic reactions ranging from hives to shock.

The type of shock we are talking about here is called anaphylaxis, and ultimately causes the person to stop breathing. Fortunately it's rare, and people that are prone usually have an EpiPen with them at all times.

An EpiPen is a device that injects epinephrine (adrenalin) under the skin, halting the runaway reaction that otherwise would lead to cardiovascular collapse. If someone is having a severe reaction, and doesn't have an EpiPen, the epinephrine that comes mixed with lidocaine will not work as a substitute. It's not nearly concentrated enough.

Mild allergic reactions leading to hives are most common. Many people know what hives look and feel like. For those who have not experienced them, they appear as raised red patches, sometimes with normal appearing skin in the center. Ringworm looks similar, but you can tell the difference by the scaly skin tissue attached to ringworms outer "ring." Also, ringworm does not come and go. This helps differentiate them from hives, which fluctuate in location and size, often hour by hour.

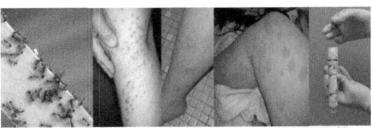

Ants both bite and sting. If a person is allergic to bees or wasps, they can also have reactions to ants. Most only get hives, some may go into shock.

Most allergic reactions are limited to hives. Some people can go into shock. These people usually know of their allergy, and carry an epinephrine pen. It's more concentrated than the epi mixed with lidocaine.

Benadryl is effective for treating hives and other allergic reactions. It's inexpensive when purchased in bulk, and like doxycycline, should be in every medical kit.

Since we are on the subject of telling hives from ringworm, a few words on the subject of skin fungi are appropriate.

Ringworm isn't a worm, it's a fungus. It's responsible for jock itch and athlete's foot. The "worm" portion of its name comes from the circular appearance of its outer scaly ring. It's quite common in people traveling through the woods, and in grim living conditions.

Sunlight kills ringworm, as it does other fungi. So don't cover these eruptions up with a bandage. Typically one contracts this illness from a carrier: usually a pet, clothing, or a contaminated surface. Ringworm can live on a countertop or door handle for up to six months. The traditional medical treatment involves antifungal creams, and the avoidance of topical steroids like cortisone. Steroid creams mask the underlying infection, and when they're stopped, the rash reappears, often out of control.

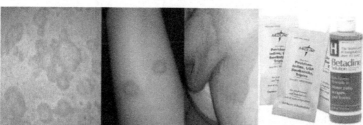

Hives. Notice there are no scales or skin flakes. Over time they will move around.

Ringworm is usually in just 1 or 2 areas, not in multiple places like hives are.

So called jock itch and athletes foot are caused by this fungus

Povidone-Iodine aka betadine, also comes in swabstick packets. They are easy to use but take up room.

Clothes and pets as well as suspicious surfaces, should be cleansed with bleach unless you're sure of the source.   Iodine has long been used as a cure, but Betadine is becoming popular.   You probably already have it in your medical kit.

SPIDERS

There are thousands of spider species, but in America only a few are harmful to humans.   The brown recluse and black widow are the biggest culprits.

Brown recluse spiders are only found in the middle United States, and only then in its southern regions.   The bites make a person ill and cause a lot of tissue damage at the bite site.   Most people suffer with nausea and fevers or chills.   Muscle aches and fatigue are common.   Severe toxicity can cause kidney failure or bleeding disorders, but this is rare.

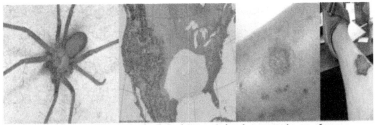

Brown recluse spiders are isolated to certain states. They can cause fever/chills, nausea and vomiting, weakness and malaise. Most damage though is done in the area of the bite, where a crater of dead tissue results.   A scarred area from a previous bite is shown on the left, a necrotic area needing debridement is shown on the right.

Black widows cause similar symptoms and are found throughout North America.   The females are more toxic than the males, but most of the damage they cause is limited to the area bitten.

It starts with a pinprick sensation, then the area turns red and swells.   Within 15 minutes to an hour, a dull cramp-like pain starts at the site, then spreads over the entire body. They can also have dizziness, trouble speaking, and anxiety. An antivenin is available, but not practical to carry into the field.

SCORPIONS

They scare hell out of many people, but few are dangerous.   Of the 1500 species found around the world, only about 25 are potentially lethal.   In America only one species, the Arizona bark scorpion, is dangerous.   Then only in very old or young people, or those with immune system impairments.

It's found in Arizona and some parts of Texas. Severe envenomation causes symptoms including seizure-like movements, paralysis, numbness and hyper-salivation. An antivenin manufactured in Mexico is available for severe cases, but its use in America is usually limited to Arizona.

All species of scorpions are able to penetrate human skin with an unpleasant sting.   With severe envenomation, symptoms can be like those of a bee or wasp sting; usually only leaving redness around stung areas.   Pain medications and cold compresses are all typically needed for treatment.

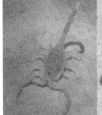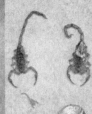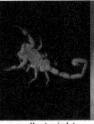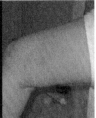

The Arizona bark scorpion is the only potentially dangerous one.	Scorpions show up well at night with a black light. Those found outside Arizona, or parts of Texas, are not dangerous to humans.	In the very old or very young, bark scorpions can kill - but usually just cause swelling.

In North America most insects, spiders, and other pesky critters are just a nuisance. Benadryl may help with the itching and swelling, ibuprofen with the pain.

The problem with any bite, poisonous or not, is it can always lead to cellulitis. The problem with cellulitis, is it can sometimes lead to flesh eating bacteria!

CELLULITIS& BACTERIA EATING FLESH

Infection of the skin, with our without an underlying abscess, is called cellulitis.   It can be lethal.

Cellulitis causes patches of skin to become red, hot and painful.   Infected areas can quickly spread to the entire extremity or face.   The disease beings when bacteria gain entry to soft tissues layers underneath the topmost layer of skin.   This usually starts by way of a cut, abrasion, or break which sometimes isn't even visible.

> *Take a ballpoint pen and outlined the infected area as soon as it appears. Every 12-24 hours re-outline the area to see if it's improving or spreading.*

Streptococcus and Staphylococcus are the most common of these bacteria, and normally live on your skin without causing problems.

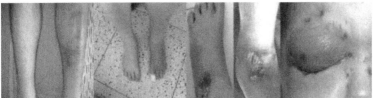

| Cellulitis often begins as small patches, then extends & produces swelling | Here the entire lower leg is affected. This will produce sepsis w/o treatment. | The burn has allowed entry of bacteria & the infection has spread quickly. | Cellulitis often involves the face and orbit. Antibiotics are required for treatment. |

Cracks in the skin, cuts, blisters, burns and insect bites can all allow entry of these bacteria to areas below the skins protective surface.   The face and lower legs are commonly affected, though the disease can occur anywhere.

Sometimes the infection will spread rapidly, and the person becomes septic quickly.   Treatment consists of resting the affected area, antibiotics, and cutting away any dead tissue.   Don't take this condition too lightly.   Rest is thought to help limit its spread, but antibiotics should be given if available.   This is one case where you might want to use two separate classes of antibiotics, especially if the infection is spreading quickly, or the patient is becoming febrile and septic.

SNAKES& DRUNKS PLAYING WITH SNAKES

Some people find them really cool, but most of us don't! Regardless, many myths surround snakes.

One important to know involves the deadliness of baby snakes. They do have more concentrated venom than adults, but only slightly. Truth be told, the bigger the snake, the more venom it's capable of injecting. Adult snakes deliver 15-20 times more poison than the young ones. And the degree of envenomation can often be correlated with its size.

Discussion of snakes in this book is limited to those found in North America, the rules here don't necessary apply to snakes found in the rest of the world. The only exception to this rule, for our purposes, are places like the everglades, where no one knows what's going on. There are Boa Constrictors and other snakes - illegally imported from the Amazon - which have been set free into the Floridian swamps. Lord only knows what's slithering around down there. If you're operating in this area, be prepared for surprises!

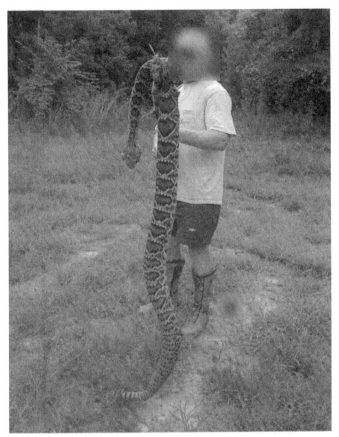

Safe Guess...
A Lot of Venom!

In the United States 25% of snake bites are dry. Meaning the person's skin has been broken, but venom hasn't been injected.   If a person doesn't have any symptoms within six or eight hours of being bitten, they will likely be fine.   At that point, only a skin infection from the puncture is a potential threat.   Antibiotics aren't necessary for prophylactic treatment.   But the wound should be cleansed with Betadine or your agent of choice. While reptile bites are famous for causing infections with the Salmonella species of bacteria, snake bites tend to cause infection with Staph, E. coli, and microbes already on your skin.

Snakes indigenous to North America come in two varieties. There are the Crotalids or pit vipers, and the Elapids, which include coral snakes.

Pit Vipers

Rattlesnakes, cottonmouths, and water moccasins derive their descriptive name from a heat sensing pit found in front of their eyes. This sensory organ allows them to gauge the amount of venom they release based on the overall heat and size of their pray.

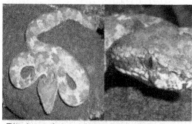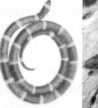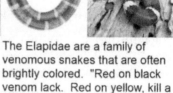

Pit vipers have triangular heads and elliptical eyes. In North America, snakes with round eyes are not poisonous. But some snakes without a triangular head, like coral snakes, are still capable of being poisonous.

The Elapidae are a family of venomous snakes that are often brightly colored. "Red on black venom lack. Red on yellow, kill a fellow."

Elapidae

This family includes snakes that are not poisonous, but brightly colored. There's an old rhyme that can help you decide if a snake is venomous: **"Red on black, venom lack. Red on yellow, kill a fellow."** With coral snakes, the red patches come in contact with yellow ones, indicating that the snake is venomous. Whereas red, black and white patched snakes, like milk snakes, are not.

The best way to prevent pit viper bites, is to stay out of areas infested with rats and small vermin. These are their primary food sources. So stay away from wood piles and compost pits. Most snake bites in the United States seem to be occurring in intoxicated people playing with them. In general there are three types of snake toxins: neurotoxins, cytotoxins, and combinations of both.

Neurotoxins are designed to slow down and immobilize the nervous system of its victim. The rodent usually doesn't get far after injection, dying of seizure and respiratory failure in minutes. Cytotoxins are essentially digestive enzymes that dissolve the pray while it's trying to run away.

In the Western United States, as you travel from north to south, the rattlesnakes go from being cytotoxic, to being neurotoxic. In the middle areas, the toxicity is mixed.

This means that a rattlesnake bite in Idaho is capable of causing tissue destruction in the bitten extremity, but doesn't cause much in the way of neurologic symptoms. When you get to Texas, effects of their bites are almost purely neurologic. Nausea and vomiting, weakness, tingling of the mouth and tongue, dizziness, muscle tremors, and altered consciousness all may result.

For the states in-between, venomous soups containing both toxins are expressed. Both cytotoxic and neurologic effects may result, but neither are as strong as snakes specializing in just one type of venom.

There are more imaginative snake bite treatments out there than hang-over cures. One of the most amusing, calls for hooking up jumper-cables to your car battery, and applying an electric shock to the bite. If you're going to apply the cables, try doing it on the snake, you'll find it much

Inner Tubes & Tourniquets

DON'T PASS UP THE OPPORTUNITY TO SCAVENGE A BICYCLE INNER TUBE. IT CAN BE CUT UP INTO STRIPS AND USED AS A LIGHT TOURNIQUET.

more rewarding!

Tourniquets come in two varieties. First, there are those aimed at completely shutting off blood flow. They're used for preventing a person from bleeding to death. The second are designed to slow but not stop blood return to the heart.

For snake bites, applying a completely constrictive tourniquet almost makes sense. But once the tourniquet is released, so is the venom... all at once. Normally your system would be exposed to it little by little, as it makes its way to your heart. This can give the body the time it needs to compensate for the effects as best possible. Releasing a constrictive tourniquet not only releases all of the poison, but all of the cellular toxins that have built up from lack of oxygen.

My favorite terrifying treatment is the old "cut the wound and suck out the poison" routine. As a cub scout, this one scared hell out of me. Not just because the thought of sucking poison out was gross, but because there was always the lingering possibility someone was seconds from getting bit on the willy. And I just knew I'd be the guy standing right next to him when it happened!

To the relief of cub scouts everywhere, this once popular treatment has fallen into disfavor. It turns out, when the skin is sliced by a blade, blood flow into the toxic tissue increases dramatically. And again the problem of too much venom getting to the heart too quickly arises.

Nowadays a very light non-constrictive tourniquet is sometimes placed, but only if the person can be transported to the hospital. Studies evaluating the effectiveness of this are lacking, and I can only offer my opinion:

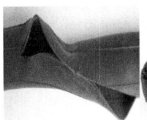 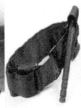 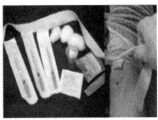

| Inner tubes have several potential uses. Making light tourniquets is just one of them. Don't ruin a good bike though, take the entire bike if you can! | This is a special tourniquet for cutting off all blood supply & can be put on with one hand. | Ordinary tourniquets only slow the venous return to the heart. They can be used for snake bites, or staring an I.V. These are not the type used to stop a person from bleeding to death. |

If the snake is likely to be neurotoxic, then I would put on a light tourniquet, a little less tight than that when you have your blood drawn. This may help slow the venom's return to the heart. If the snakes cytotoxic, I would just elevate the extremity. In this instance, I would want the poison to disseminate in hopes of diluting it a little at the site.

Conventional medicine treats venomous snake bites with antivenin. When available it's the treatment of choice for both Crotalids and Elapids.

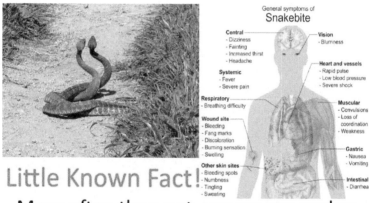

General symptoms of
Snakebite

Central
- Dizziness
- Fainting
- Increased thirst
- Headache

Systemic
- Fever
- Severe pain

Respiratory
- Breathing difficulty

Wound site
- Bleeding
- Fang marks
- Discoloration
- Burning sensation
- Swelling

Other skin sites
- Bleeding spots
- Numbness
- Tingling
- Sweating

Vision
- Blurriness

Heart and vessels
- Rapid pulse
- Low blood pressure
- Severe shock

Muscular
- Convulsions
- Loss of coordination
- Weakness

Gastric
- Nausea
- Vomiting

Intestinal
- Diarrhea

Little Known Fact!
More often than not, venomous snakes travel in Pairs!   -ThePrepperPages.com

COTTONMOUTHS, WATER MOCCASINS, AND CORAL SNAKES

None of these make good pets. They deliver potent neurotoxins, but only a few in North America are toxic. People get very sick when bitten. Symptoms mimic those of neurotoxic rattle snakes. Antivenin is the treatment of choice... if available.   Otherwise immobilize the limb and provide "supportive care."   Supportive care, in this case, might involve smoking the herbal remedies you've swiped from your neighbor's kid's rooms earlier.   The anxiety of having to wait and see just how bad the toxin is going to suck can be enormous.

Now let's turn our attention now to something that doesn't bite... plants!

PLANTS FROM HELL – POISON IVY, OAK & SUMAC

As a prepper, you're likely familiar with the horrors of poison ivy, oak and sumac. And you can probably avoid them most of the time. But in the darkness of night, accidently brushing against a plant while out on patrol, or worse, when using the "facilities" - *is not uncommon.*

If you know you've been exposed, you can wash the slippery resin off your skin in time. But most never realize their trespass, and only learn of it 12-72 hours later when blisters begin forming. By that time it's too late. The oily resin on the underside of the leaves has now firmly attached to your skin. After 30 minutes, there's no way to remove it. It must fall off on its own - *and that takes three weeks.* Symptoms are most severe on days four through seven.

The oil can rub off you and onto your pets, clothes, bedding and friends during this period. You end up sharing the itchy, swollen, red rash and its weeping blisters with others. That being said, the poison is rarely spread from one person's skin to another's after it's been washed with soap. Further, if the blisters break open, the fluid will not contaminate other people.

The itch-inducing resin in all three plants is Urushiol. It's an oil that's contained in the plants' roots, stems, and leaves. It sticks to anything it touches. If your dog rubs up against you after he's brushed against one of the plants, you end up with a rash. Worse yet, if someone is burning the plants and you're close by, the resin can aerosolize and land on your skin.

You'll know the rash is from poison ivy, oak, or sumac because of its linear chain of blisters, something you'd expect after brushing past one of the leafs. When aerosolized, this rule no longer holds true, and blisters are randomly spread over areas not covered by clothing.

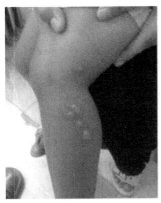
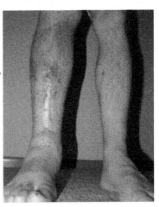

Left: linear blisters of poison ivy.

Right: diffuse blisters & swelling aerosolized contact.

Poison ivy, oak, and sumac all have a three leaf design at the end of their stems. All grow in most regions of the country. And all carry the Urushiol oil or resin. In each case it sticks to a surface for a month before falling off. Once the rash appears, the sap like substance can't be washed off. Right after contact, it's believed the oil can be removed with soapy water or alcohol, but only if you get to it within the first 30 minutes.

POISON IVY

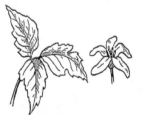

Poison ivy can be a shrub or an ivy. Note the end leaf structures.

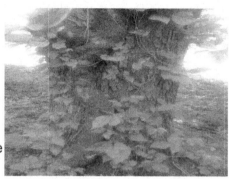

The features of this plant are its green pointed leaves hanging from the stem in groups of three. It grows as a shrub or a vine, and its appearance changes with the seasons. Yellow-green flowers are seen in the spring, and change to yellow-red in autumn. Typically it grows along river banks in the form of a vine.

POISON OAK

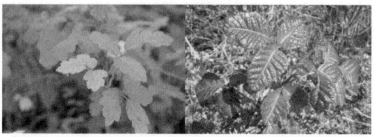

Poison oak can be a shrub or vine. Its leafs look a little like oak leafs and turn color in the fall. Note the 3 leaf structure.

Much like poison ivy, poison oak leaves also cluster in sets of three. The edges of the solid green leaves look a little bit like condensed leaves of an oak tree. Most often seen in shrub form, it can also be a vine, and is mostly found on the West Coast.

POISON SUMAC

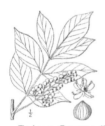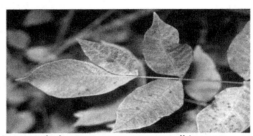

Poison Sumac likes to grow in boggy areas as a small tree or shrub. Note the 3 leaf structure is not always an exact rule in every single stem. Nature can do this, so check several stems.

Usually growing as a small tree or shrub, sumac loves boggy areas and is usually found in swamps. Poison sumac leafs are packed with Urushiol, so much so they produce black or brownish-black spots. Leaf stems contain 7-13 leaflets arranged in pairs, and grow abundantly along the Mississippi River.

TREATMENT & MANAGEMENT

One of the most important things to do, is to scrub under your fingernails to prevent the resin from spreading to areas you're unconsciously scratching.

Treating Poison Ivy, Oak, and Sumac

o In minor cases, calamine lotion and hydrocortisone cream can help with the itching and blistering. Benadryl may also be used.

o Sweating aggravates the itching, so try to stay cool and apply cool compresses to your skin.

o Bathing in warm water with an oatmeal bath has been used for years, its effectiveness remains uncertain.

o Bathe animals to remove the resin from their fur.

o Wash the clothing and the shoes involved, with soap and hot water.

o For severe cases, steroids pills like prednisone may be used - if available.

Never burn poison ivy, oak, or sumac. While the aerosolized resin may cause a terrible rash, inhaling it will cause potentially lethal blisters in the lungs.

THORNS AND CACTUS

Other troublesome but unrelated plants are those with thorns or needles. Both can evoke an inflammatory reaction and cause intense itching. The best way to remove the needles, is to pour rubber cement over the area and wait for it to harden. Then peel it back and the needles will come out with it. Duct tape works as a substitute.

249

Remember this because most of us don't carry rubber cement around. Duct tape... that's is a different story.

Eating unfamiliar plants as a food source is always risky.

Rubber Cement

KEEP AN EYE OUT FOR RUBBER CEMENT IN YOUR TRAVELS. IT'S NOT A HIGH PRIORITY ITEM, UNLESS YOU'RE IN A DESERT ENVIRONMENT, THEN YOU'LL NEED IT FOR REMOVING CACTUS NEEDLES.

Over 75% are toxic to humans. The other day while lecturing, I was asked why humans taste bitterness. After all, few people enjoy the flavor. It's probably because organic toxins often taste bitter. This may have evolved as an evolutionary defense mechanism, one discouraging us from eating poison plants. You've probably already experienced this when taking aspirin. It's made from willow bark, and very bitter if you don't swallow it right away. For humans aspirin is only toxic in large doses, but the principle is the same. The reflex to spit out bitter tasting plants may have aided in our early efforts at survival.

Next up: Fish and the drugs they love!

SECTION FOUR

DEALING WITH COMMON BUT DEADLY INFECTIONS & CONDITIONS

YES, YOU AND YOUR FISH CAN TAKE THE SAME PILLS "FISH-I-CILLIN"

Preppers anguish over antibiotics. They tend to be concerned with their availability after a collapse. Hopefully this chapter will dissolve those worries. Like narcotics, the value of antibiotics is known intrinsically to just about everyone. Both are just about as valuable in bartering, as in health. But they can be hard to come by. Buying them overseas through the internet is easy, but sometimes prohibitively expensive.

In past years the best way to get Ciprofloxin, or any other antibiotic, was from your doctor. They'll usually prescribe antibiotics and antidiarrheals if you're traveling overseas, and might get sick. But only one course of treatment is typically dispensed. And the bottle they're in is rarely air sealed. Recently I've seen physicians in America advertising for services where they will write the prescriptions for you through the mail. I don't know how long big brother is going to put up with that. The DEA gets real snippety when it learns of such proposals. For most people, fish antibiotics will be the best way to go.

Fish and bird antibiotics are a hot topic on the internet lately. People want to know if they're suitable as a substitute for people. The potential liability for answering "yes" is obvious. But that liability works both ways.

Fish Pills

MORE PRODUCTIVE THAN RUMMAGING THROUGH A PHARMACY, IS SEARCHING A PET STORE. LOOTERS ARE LESS LIKELY TO HIT A TROPICAL FISH STORE THAN A RITE-AID. LOOK FOR FISH-FLOX (CIPROFLOXIN), FISH-MOX (AMOXICILLIN), FISH-ZOLE (METRONIDAZOLE), FISH-SULFA (SULFAMETHOXAZOLE / TRIMETHOPRIM) AND BIRD BIOTIC (DOXYCYCLINE.)

The fish pills I've seen come in capsules marked with numbers. Many times the color of the capsule, and the numbers imprinted on it, are identical to the human variety when matched side by side (I'm using the Physicians Desktop Reference {PDR} for the comparison.) This is where the liability issue works in your favor.

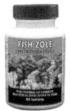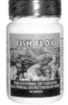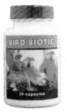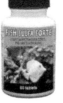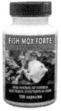

Flagyl (for Giardia)   Ciprofloxin   Doxycycline   Bactrim DS   Amoxicillin

Imagine for a moment that a guy working at a fish store was prescribed Amoxicillin by his doctor, and had it filled at the local Wall-Mart. Now he's at work and accidently spills his pills in with the ones he was supposed to give to the fish later that day. He tries to separate out his, only to find it's impossible; both are marked the same. Figuring there must be no difference, he takes one... but then has a reaction. Who is legally liable? Everyone. The pharmaceutical company is liable, so is the dispensing pharmacy.

It may go without saying, but only take fish antibiotics if human pills are not available!

While this is an unlikely scenario, risk management divisions within large pharmaceutical companies are no joke. They're unlikely to have overlooked the possibility something like this could occur, however improbable.

These companies are used to getting blindsided, they do everything possible to avoid it.

If the pet antibiotics are marked exactly as those in the PDR, then personally I believe they are the same. From the manufacturing plant they must be shipping some to the animal division, and the rest to the human side for packaging and distribution.

Fish and bird antibiotics have the advantage of coming in sealed containers, and likely have longer practical shelf lives than those dispensed from a pharmacy.

As long as society is intact, take people pills. When it unravels, steal from the fish!

PREPPER EYE PROBLEMS

Pink eye and corneal abrasions are among the most common ocular conditions encountered in the field.

Eye injuries and infections can be as disabling to a zombie prepper as a broken arm or leg. Debris from disasters often stays suspended in the atmosphere for hours to days. Recall those images of 9/11, and you'll see why it's important to feel comfortable treating these conditions. Those of concern to preppers fall into two categories: pink eye and corneal abrasions.

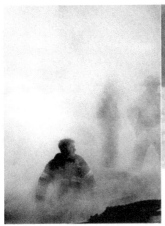
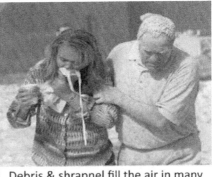

Debris & shrapnel fill the air in many disasters. Even when people have eye protection they don't think to use it.

PINK EYE

This is a catch all label referring to just about any type of ocular infection. Typically it's caused by a virus, though rarely bacteria can be responsible. At first the infection feels like a scratch or abrasion, or like it does when you have something in your eye. Over the next hours to days, the white part of the eye - the sclera - becomes reddened from inflamed blood vessels which are normally invisible. Goopy eyes may follow. But infection isn't the only cause of an ocular discharge. Corneal abrasions can produce the same picture, even if infection isn't present.

CORNEAL ABRASIONS

Scratches of the eye occur when the clear part of the eye, the cornea, sustains a minor abrasion but produces major pain and tearing that can limit vision.

Corneal abrasions occur when the clear part of the eye, the cornea, sustains a minor scratch but produces major pain and tearing. We discussed this injury earlier, and said that patching for 24 hours is generally all that's needed for its resolution.

Physicians will sometimes stain the eye with fluorescein, a dye which is taken up by the scratched area, and reveals the percentage of cornea damaged. If greater than 50%, the patch should be left on for 48 hours instead of 24. Because the dye won't be available to us, you'll have to decide on symptoms alone. So injuries consistent with larger abrasions should be patched for two days instead of one.

Physicians will sometimes stain the eye with a dye called fluorescein. It comes on a strip that looks like litmus paper and is touched to the sclera. The person then blinks a few times and the dye spreads out over the eye.

If a scratch is present the dye will be taken up by the injured area, and a green line will appear revealing the location and percentage of cornea damaged. If the dye is not taken up, the doctor assumes the cause of the problem is infection.

While you may have eye patches in your medical kit, the dye won't likely be available. So the best strategy for preppers is to remember a treatment that will work for both conditions.

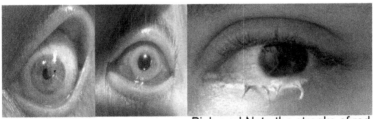

Scratched eye, stained to take up green dye.

Looks bad but is harmless. Sub-conjunctival bleed

Pink eye! Note the streaks of red over the white area (sclera) and the watery to puss like discharge.

In an ideal world the treatment of either problem might involve anti-inflammatory eye drops; sometimes with antibiotics mixed in. Eye irrigation to remove foreign debris and irritants should also be considered. The problem for the prepper is that neither will likely be available. So patching the eye for a few days is the best that can be done.

If you don't have any eye patches in your kit, cut a gauze into an oval shape. Have the person close their eye, then tape or somehow secure the patch in place. In 24 hours most eye abrasions will heal if covered. And within two days most ocular infections will resolve.

Take home message: In a disaster situation when you're not sure of if it's an infection or an abrasion causing the eye symptoms, treat the person as if they have both. Wash it out if you can, then patch it for 48 hours.

Treatment involves anti-inflammatory eye drops, sometimes with antibiotics mixed in. These probably won't be available in times of global disaster, so patching the eye for a few days is the best that can be done. Wearing cotton gloves can help remind the person not to touch their eye, and inadvertently spread the disease to others.

SUBCONJUNCTIVAL HEMORRHAGES

These look horrific... *but are harmless*. Often resulting from the most minor of traumas, including coughing, the white sclera becomes completely red. One of the blood vessels running between the clear covering of the eye and the white sclera breaks open. A very small amount of blood spreads out encircling the cornea. It will change colors like a bruise before resolving in the following weeks.

Side Note: How to Tell if Your Neighbor Has Ebola From Across the Street

(This section is included here, because in an apocalypse, the only way you'll be able to tell if a person has Ebola, is by looking for specific changes in a person's sclera and skin.)

Ebola belongs to a group of viruses made of four families which produce a fatal illness called Viral Hemorrhagic Fever.   We're using Ebola as an example here, but the signs and symptoms are common to them all.

You'll probably want to be able to tell if they're infected from a distance - way across the street preferably! So we've developed the following checklist:

FIRST... ARE THEY IN BED AND BARFING?

If so, they might have Ebola.

After glancing at the symptoms in the box, recall your last flu-like illness, and compare those symptoms with the ones listed. With exception of the "unexplained bleeding or bruising" – which is a late finding in Ebola – they're similar to those caused by many common infectious illnesses.

WEST AFRICA
Ebola Outbreak

Early Symptoms:

Ebola can only be spread to others after symptoms begin. Symptoms can appear from 2 to 21 days after exposure.

- Fever
- Headache
- Diarrhea
- Vomiting
- Stomach pain
- Muscle pain
- Unexplained bleeding or bruising

SECOND... DO THEY HAVE A FEVER?

Since you're across the street, just look to see if they're all sweaty - or ask someone that's closer!

Fever is always thought to be present with Ebola... always!   But alone, an elevated body temperature is hardly specific for the disease.   That's because fever is the rule with most viral infections, not the exception.   So using that sign to try to sort out Ebola patients from those having the flu for example - *is pointless.*   It only tells you the person is coming down with an illness.   Not which one.

THIRD... ARE THEY COUGHING?

If so, shucks, they probably don't have Ebola.

Ebola rarely produces a cough, whereas influenza frequently does.   But most telling of those stricken with Ebola, is the unusual skin rash, and a specific type of redness in the whites of their eyes that appear.   Most of the time the skin and eye findings show up before the person starts vomiting blood.   If they are bleeding from every orifice, then Ebola, or another virus from its family, is more or less certain.

FOURTH... NO COUGH?

Well Then Cowboy, You'll Have to Sneak Close Enough to See the Whites of Their Eyes!

Ebola does something strange to the eyes. The whites of their eyes become a bizarre type of red. Normally this is called conjunctivitis, and is found with many contagious illness. But in the case of Ebola the redness is distinctly different. It's deeper and reflects processes occurring in all vessels of the body. Because this is an important finding, we'll delve into it a little more carefully. Let's start with what the whites of normal eyes should look like.

262

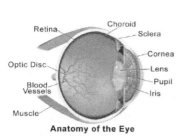

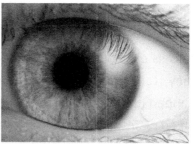

Retina, Choroid, Sclera, Cornea, Lens, Pupil, Iris, Optic Disc, Blood Vessels, Muscle

Anatomy of the Eye

Covering the white part of the eye (sclera) is a transparent & movable layer (conjunctiva) containing blood vessels. A few blood vessels are seen normally & are mobile with a Q-Tip.

All of these findings are common to many non-fatal viral illnesses. Their typical appearance is shown in the images below.

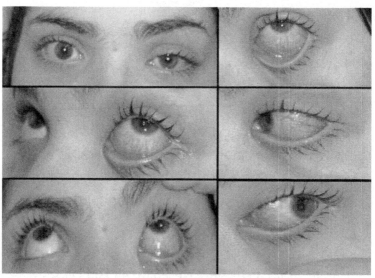

Conjunctivitis like you'd see with someone who has the flu. Notice how the blood vessels are pointing toward the pupil in a radial pattern, & not running circumferentially around it.

The redness Ebola produces is different. The blood vessel damage is seen deep within the whitened area.

Vessels there will not move or blanch when you push on them. This is bad news, because it suggests that blood vessels elsewhere in the body aren't just irritated, but that they too are sustaining massive injury. And if that's happening in the eye, then the person is probably close to bleeding into all of their organs. Even without manipulating the eye with a Q-Tip, you'll notice the inflamed vessels aren't traveling in the usual radial direction. Instead, they're running circumferentially around the iris.

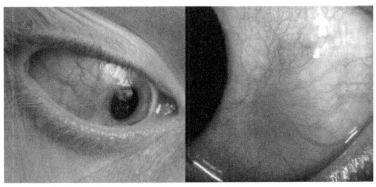

With Ebola, the blood vessels being damaged are deep within the sclera, and aren't movable with a Q-Tip, or blanchable when you push down on them - like they are with conjunctivitis caused by the flu.

LAST... DO THEY HAVE BLOOD BLISTERS?

You didn't want to get close enough to see the whites of their eyes, you say? Can't blame you! In that case wait a bit. In the last stages you'll be able to see the Ebola rash from across the street.

The rash Ebola produces is unique. Where most rashes result from skin inflammation, the hemorrhagic rash of Ebola results from bleeding into the skin. In addition, these non-blanching purplish spots cover most of the person's body, not just a specific area.

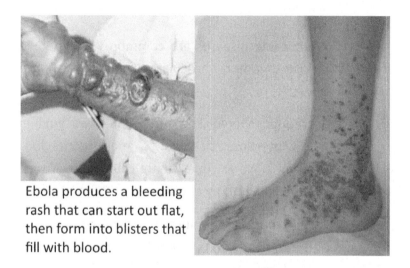

Ebola produces a bleeding rash that can start out flat, then form into blisters that fill with blood.

Now you know they have Ebola... or Marburg - Any of the 4 families of virus that cause Viral Hemorrhagic Fever

As Ebola progresses, the symptoms become more telling and appear in a predictable sequence. About half of those infected will go on to bleed internally. This effect is common with Marburg and Filoviruses (Ebola), and the Viral Hemorrhagic Fever they cause.

COLDS, SORE THROATS, & COMMON INFECTIONS

Rule 44- *"First things first, hide the women and children"* - Leroy Jethro Gibbs, NCIS

Communicable diseases are common when people are packed close together, particularly in the late fall into deep winter.

The prepper should keep in mind two guiding principles of wintertime sickness: most contagious illnesses occurring in North America are caused by viruses, and viruses aren't killed off by antibiotics.

The black plague and cholera may reappear in Europe and parts of the third world, but hopefully won't surface in America. Viral infections like Measles, Mumps, and Rubella are also unlikely to become a threat. Most of us and our children have been immunized.

Washing your hands and coughing into your elbow crease do more to prevent infections, than wearing surgical masks or isolating people with minor illness. Most of the viruses we are talking about are either spread by contact with an infected surface, or are airborne and carried by respiratory droplets. This is why soap and water and correct coughing technique are so important.

Most colds and flu will appear after the initial stress of the disaster is over, and preppers have settled down and into a routine. The general stress a person is under until then, winds up the immune system and protects them for as long as possible. However this is a debt that eventually must be paid back. Illness becomes more prevalent at this stage.

SORE THROATS

Most people get these from time to time, especially if they have small children in public schools. Kids are walking petri dishes, often bringing germs home for everyone's enjoyment. Most causes are viral, but can sometimes be bacterial.

Medicine has struggled with how and when to treat sore throats for the past 50 years, but finally a global recommendation has been made: even if the sore throat is caused by bacteria, it should not be treated with antibiotics, unless it's strep.

Studies have clearly been shown **not** to speed the person's recovery. The exception is strep throat. But it's not treated to help the person get better, it's treated to reduce the incidence of related diseases that streptococcus can cause. Scarlet fever, rheumatic fever, post-streptococcal glomerular nephritis (inflammation of the kidneys,) even nervous tics and movement disorders can all result from a strep infection. This is why when you bring the kids to the doctors for a sore throat, they do a rapid strep test in the office. If it's negative, antibiotics aren't prescribed.

In the field it might be wise to give the person amoxicillin, as rapid strep tests are not going to be available. Remember to ask the person if they are allergic to penicillin beforehand. Allergic reactions usually result in skin rashes, but in rare cases a type of shock called anaphylaxis can occur.

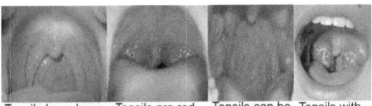

Tonsils have been removed. Mildly inflamed throat. Tonsils are red & inflamed. No puss is seen. Tonsils can be small but spread around. Tonsils with exudate or puss.

When you look into someone's throat, you may find they've had their tonsils removed, but they can still get strep and other types of infections. Tonsils are really aggregates of small lymph nodes, and some people have more than others (shown in the third picture to the right.) Unfortunately you can't tell what's causing the infection:

virus, strep, or another bacteria.   Not from its appearance alone.

Finally, remember that children younger than two don't get strep.   The bacteria can't adhere to the throat without a special protein receptor the child makes.   That doesn't happen until they're about two-and-a-half years old.

Smoke is never a stranger when apocalypse is throwing the party.   Veterans returning from the 1991 Gulf War have tried to explain to me what it's like when oil wells are set afire.   But they'd always say their words were inadequate.   The smell of war is apparently something one must experience to understand.   All mucus membranes sting relentlessly, and the work of breathing at rest is incredible.   Sinus and lung infections cannot help themselves in these conditions - they will hunt you down till you're found.

Let's turn our attention to preventing and treating these monsters now!

THE MYSTERY OF SINUSITIS

Apocalyptic smoke from burning buildings and smoldering zombie corpuses ensures that sinusitis will be a major problem facing preppers.   It is a predictable manifestation of the death and destruction inseparable from war and catastrophe, and one common to those caught up in WWII.

It's the headaches mixed with profound congestion making these infections so enjoyable.   Add-in the difficulty breathing, from accompanying bronchitis or pneumonia, and you get a knock-out punch capable of bringing well planned bug-outs to a screeching halt.   Traveling over land with a head cold is a type of misery best avoided.   Most attempts at warding off the monster fail.   Particularly in times like The Gulf War, when the smoke from burning oil wells never seemed to clear.

HOW DO YOU TREAT SINUSITIS?

It's more difficult than you might imagine.   You see, we still aren't really sure what it is.   Let me explain:

The sinuses air-filled bony cavities lined with a mucus producing tissue.   Essentially, they're a system of labyrinths that ultimately connect and drain through your nose. The mucus of the sinuses collect bacteria inhaled throughout the day, then tries to flush them out like the lungs do - only from above. Normally drained by gravity, these cavities don't always empty – not in humans anyway.

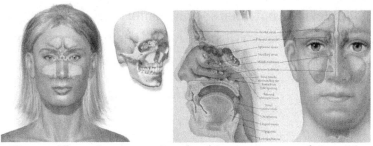

The maxillary sinuses are involved in most cases of sinusitis. Note the upward location & direction of the drainage routes.

The fundamental problem is illustrated above. Notice in human drainage canals, the exit conduits leading from the bony cavities are orientated *upward*. They're having to drain *against* gravity. Thought to be a consequence of standing upright, once we climbed down from the trees, the illness is mostly one of people and rarely seen in animals.

Four-legged critters have a head orientation rotated 90 degrees downward from ours. An orientation we have only when looking down at our shoes. This allows an animal's sinuses to drain with the help of gravity 24 hours a day. For us, only when we sleep do we assume a gravity favoring posture. But even then the direction is horizontal and less than optimal.

Suspect you have a sinus infection if your head cold just won't go away. Particularly if accompanied by fevers or chills. Other symptoms include a dull ache or pressure in your forehead that's worse when looking down. Pushing with your fingers over the sinuses in attempt to elicit tenderness has not been shown helpful in telling if you have sinusitis. Without a CT scan, you'll have to go on symptoms alone.

> *Nasal rinses work best when given early in the course of a sinus infection. To make your own rinse, add 1/4 tsp of salt to 8 oz. of warm water. Adding ¼ tsp of baking soda to the mix can help sooth swollen nasal passages.*

Acute sinusitis can last up to a month, but what role bacteria play, if any, has been debated for years and is still unknown.

There are two main reasons that antibiotics are generally not given for this condition, or at least not for the first two weeks: First, we are not sure that even chronic cases of sinusitis have a bacterial cause.

Second, if it is bacterial, we think they are coating themselves with a protective biofilm, making them almost inaccessible to the immune system and antibiotics.

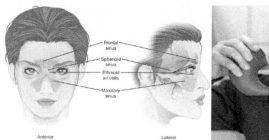 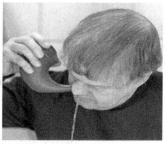

Nasal washes are a brutal cure, but they work. Mix up your solution, lean your head forward, and rinse 2-3 times a day. Add baking soda to decrease nasal swelling.

Biofilms are complex aggregates of other bacterial species that surround and protect the evil-doers. In animal models, biofilms have been shown to increase the bacteria's resistance to antibiotics by one-thousand fold. Meaning even if they are in there, they'll be chuckling at your amoxicillin as it floats by. Better to thin the mucus with lots of water and let nature deal with the matter. You'll want to be patient, because it takes months to resolve in certain instances - *like when you cannot escape the smoke.*

EAR INFECTIONS

As with pink eye and sore throats, ear infections are usually self-limiting; meaning they'll resolve on their own without treatment. The reason we're considering all three, is because they make children cry. Military history is full of heartbreaking stories where children have given away the position of those hiding; and of little ones suffocated by their parents to prevent it from happening.

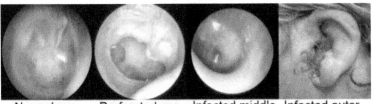

| Normal ear drum. No infection. | Perforated ear drum. Do not use lidocaine. | Infected middle ear. Note redness and puss. | Infected outer ear. Note the puss on outside |

MIDDLE EAR INFECTIONS

While you probably won't be looking in the ears of children, an infection can be presumed if the little rascal is fussy and tugging on their earlobe.   Most parents have sat up with a child all night because ear infections are so painful. But there's a solution.   It's unapproved and unconventional... *but it works.*

If the child does not have ear tubes, or a suspected perforation of their eardrum, you can drop lidocaine into the ear canal while they lay on their side.   Insert a cotton ball or foam hearing protector to help keep the anesthetic in. Mixing lidocaine with long acting bupivacaine can extend the pain relief for up to six hours.   The anesthetics numb pain receptors on the eardrum, allowing everyone to sleep, or at least keep quiet in times of trouble.

This treatment should not be used if there's a hole in the eardrum, either from a perforation, or from an ear tube. The lidocaine will get into the middle ear where small bones transmitting sound are located. The medication may injure or even dissolve these structures.

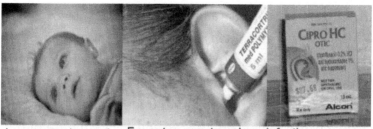

In emergencies, and if you're sure the eardrum is intact, drop lidocaine in to numb the typanic membrane.

For outer, or external ear infections, you can make up something similar to cipro drops by mixing Fish Flox in saline or lidocaine. Or you can use a topical antibiotic, and place it in the external ear canal.

Amoxicillin can be used for treating middle ear infections, but as with most antibiotics, bacterial resistance to the drug can be high.

EXTERNAL EAR INFECTIONS

When you see crusting or puss like material coming out of the ear, the infection is probably not in the middle ear, but in the external canal. It can be from the middle ear, but only if the eardrum has ruptured releasing the material. In this case the person commonly has some degree of pain relief, as the pressure causing the pain has been normalized. External ear infections usually cause swelling you can see, helping tell the difference between outer and middle ear infections. Adults typically get external ear infections, whereas middle ear infections are the domain of children.

DIZZINESS AND VERTIGO

The next consideration of ear troubles involves one of the scariest conditions... vertigo. Colds and other conditions can cause inflammation in the balance centers of the inner ear. You may feel fine, then without warning, the world literally starts spinning. You lose your balance and become nauseated. The sudden and severe nature of this condition might make you think you're having a stroke, or that you have a brain tumor.

The anxiety this produces can uncouple you, especially in the context of the apocalypse. The good news is that the worse the symptoms, the less likely it's anything serious. Tumors grow slowly producing symptoms over time. Strokes can cause similar symptoms, but are rare and usually accompanied by other obvious neurological symptoms. While symptoms can last several weeks, they diminish and disappear over time.

Let's look now at common infections that will kill you long before the zombies have a chance!

INFECTIONS & CONDITIONS THAT OCCLUDE THE UPPER AIRWAY

Three life-threatening conditions commonly occlude the upper airway, and they can all produce a high-pitched whistling sound called stridor.

Stridor

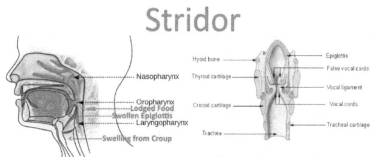

Stridor is a high-pitched musical breath sound caused by turbulent air flow in the upper airway. Often you can hear it without a stethoscope. There are 3 common causes: Airway swelling from Croup, Epiglottitis, & lodged foreign bodies.

The first cause of stridor is from some type of foreign object the child has tried to swallow, but has gotten stuck in their airway. Legos are infamous for this. Sometimes you can carefully sneak in and extract it. Other times you can't. Fortunately, they're relatively rare. You'll have to get them to cough or drool it out.

Our image about stridor in the previous page shows the location of the epiglottis and larynx. Both can swell rapidly from infections, quickly narrowing their airway. This can happen faster than you might imagine. Let's look into the specifics of these illnesses. There are several, but the potentially life-threatening ones are epiglottitis and croup.

EPIGLOTTITIS & THE 4 D'S

The epiglottis is a type of "tissue gate" located above the vocal cords. Normally it prevents food from going down your trachea and into your lungs when you're swallowing. We don't know why, but sometimes it can become infected and rapidly swell shut.

Most of us were taught in medical school that epiglottitis is a disease of childhood, but George Washington probably died from it - and he wasn't a spring chicken.

The infection is caused by a bacteria with a misleading name - Haemophilus influenzae. This bacterium was mistakenly considered to be the source of influenza until 1933. Only then was it learned "the flu" is actually caused by a virus.

We've been vaccinating children against this bacterium's most prevalent form, H. influenzae type b, since the mid to late 1990s. You may recognize it on your child's immunization records by the acronym Hib. While less

278

prevalent than before, other strains of the species continue to cause problems in all recesses of the world.

You might first suspect a child has this illness when you hear stridor, but usually there are additional findings. Known as the "4 D's," the presence of these signs and symptoms help confirm your suspicion of epiglottitis.

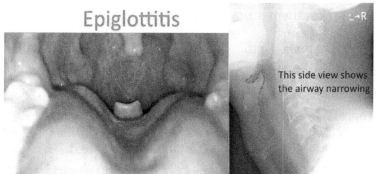

Epiglottitis

This side view shows the airway narrowing

George Washington was thought to have died of epiglottitis. Untreated, this bacterial infection can be fatal in children. As swelling increases, the airway narrows causing the "4 D's." Dyspnea (shortness of breath), respiratory Distress, Difficulty swallowing & Drooling

The Four D's of Epiglottitis	What You'll See & Hear
#1 Drooling	The child cannot swallow their secretions, so they just drool!
#2 Dysphagia	Medical term for having difficulty swallowing
#3 Dyspnea	Medical term for having difficulty breathing, and being short of breath (SOB)

| #4 Distress | They appear scared - they know something is terribly wrong, and often start to panic |

Typically the child will be leaning forward and Drooling copiously. They'll either have Difficulty swallowing (known as Dysphagia in medicine), or not be able to swallow at all. The difficulty or inability to swallow is what makes them drool and lean forward.

Dyspnea is the medical term for having difficulty breathing and being short of breath (SOB). This finding is troubling. It suggests the person's airway is undergoing progressive and accelerated closure. It' swelling shut!

Our 4th and final D stands for Distress. These children look scared and panicky. Some instinctual part of them knows they're in trouble. They'll often be totally focused on trying to catch their breath. Their appearance can range from extremely anxious, like you'd see with a drowning person, to completely exhausted. It's an ugly scene all around!

Visualize for a moment a pipe or cardboard tube representing the child's airway. Now imagine the inside wall of the tube thickening inward by ¼ of an inch. This small amount of narrowing is minor at first. But with the second ¼ inch of swelling, the lumen will effectively narrow twice what it did the first time. This is why airway occlusion progresses so rapidly.

Antibiotics will be needed for this infection, and they should be started as soon as possible.   Ideally you'd give intravenous antibiotics, but that's unlikely to be available in the conditions you're going to be up against.

All-in-all it's a hardy bug.   Resistance to penicillin is the rule, not the exception.   The only penicillin type antibiotics likely to work, are those with a combination of ampicillin and sulbactam.   This combination is known by the trade name Augmentin.   Though generic equivalents are much cheaper and easier to come by.   Just look for an antibiotic with both "ampicillin" and "sulbactam" or "clavulanate" printed on the bottle.

The dosage for adults is one 875-mg every 12 hours, or if you have the 500-mg tablets, one tablet every 8 hours. The dose for children weighing 40 kg (88 lbs.) is the same as for adults.   For ages 3 months and up use the following table:

Augmentin Dosing in Children & Adults

INFECTION	DOSING REGIMEN	
	EVERY 12 HOURS	EVERY 8 HOURS
	200 MG/5 ML OR 400 MG/5 ML ORAL SUSPENSION[A]	125 MG/5 ML OR 250 MG/5 ML ORAL SUSPENSION[A]
Otitis media[b], sinusitis, lower respiratory tract infections, and more severe infections	45 mg/kg/day every 12 hours	40 mg/kg/day every 8 hours
Less severe infections	25 mg/kg/day every 12 hours	20 mg/kg/day every 8 hours

[a]Each strength of suspension of AUGMENTIN is available as a chewable tablet for use by older children.

[b]Duration of therapy studied and recommended for acute otitis media is 10 days.

Adopted with permission from: www.rxlist.com/augmentin-drug/indications-dosage.htm

Another good choice is Cipro (Ciprofloxacin). But this is almost never the first choice of physicians when treating children. Early on there were reported side effects in ages 1-17. But that fear has lessened considerably in the last couple decades. It's safe enough that I'd give it to my children if Augmentin didn't work or wasn't available.

One of the advantages of Cipro in general, is the many types of infections it can be used to treat – even for treating people exposed to anthrax. A table of its uses and dosages is in the appendix of this book. For now, the dosing breaks down as follows:

Cipro (Ciprofloxacin) Dosing for Adults

INFECTION	ADULT DOSAGE GUIDELINES			
	SEVERITY	DOSE	FREQUENCY	USUAL DURATIONS†
Urinary Tract	Acute Uncomplicated	250 mg	q 12 h	3 days
	Mild/Moderate	250 mg	q 12 h	7 to 14 days
	Severe/ Complicated	500 mg	q 12 h	7 to 14 days
Chronic Bacterial Prostatitis	Mild/ Moderate	500 mg	q 12 h	28 days
Lower Respiratory Tract	Mild/ Moderate	500 mg	q 12 h	7 to 14 days
	Severe/ Complicated	750 mg	q 12 h	7 to 14 days
Acute Sinusitis	Mild/ Moderate	500 mg	q 12 h	10 days
Skin and	Mild/ Moderate	500 mg	q 12 h	7 to 14 days
Skin Structure	Severe/ Complicated	750 mg	q 12 h	7 to 14 days

With permission: www.rxlist.com/cipro-drug/indications-dosage.htm

For children the dosage is 10 to 20 mg/kg every 12 hours. So versatile is Cipro for nearly all the infections a prepper is likely to get – respiratory, gastrointestinal, and skin – it's one of the four antibiotics I carry in my medical bag.

Before we move on, please note that in addition to antibiotics, patients with epiglottitis may need steroids like prednisone to decrease the swelling. Otherwise their airway might completely close off. Typically steroids are not given to people with infections, especially when they're bacterial. They suppress the immune system and can make the infection become worse – *rapidly*!

With severe epiglottitis, when there is absolutely no chance you can get to a hospital, you may not have much choice but to use them. If the edema does not resolve, the person may die from it.

Saying "yes" to steroids, and how to dose them will be covered in the next chapter. For now, let's see the next potentially fatal infection of preppers – croup.

CROUP & BARKING SEALS

Epiglottitis can be identified by the 4 D's. With croup, by its characteristic "seal-like" barking cough.

Croup!

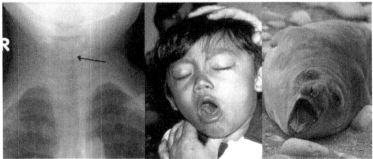

Croup is a viral infection that occurs in children. It causes stridor as the inflamed upper airway narrows (arrow). Parents can easily recognize it by the "seal-like" barking cough it produces.

Recall that viruses cannot be killed, because they aren't living organisms. So antibiotics are useless in treating viral infections.

Croup is an infection of the trachea and larynx caused by Human Parainfluenza Virus. The airway swelling it produces can be severe. Since antibiotics won't work, limiting and reversing the upper airway edema with aid of steroids is often all one can do. But that's only if the swelling is severe, and it looks like the child might begin to have trouble breathing. We still hate to use steroids when someone has a viral infection, but when compared with bacterial infections, the risk is far lower.

Prednisone is the best steroid medication to use in the field. It's also indispensable in the treatment of severe allergic reactions, and life-threatening asthma. We highly recommend carrying it in your medical kit.

If there were ever a true rescue Medicine for emergencies, it would have to be Prednisone. We strongly encourage you acquire some for your preps. Now let's talk about how and when to use it!

PREDNISONE DOSES FOR TREATING ASTHMA, SEVERE ALLERGIC REACTIONS & AIRWAY EDEMA

Age	Acute or Maintenance Tx=Treatments	Dosage
< I year	Acute	10 mg orally every 12 hours.
1 to 4 years	Acute	20 mg orally every 12 hours.
5 to 12 years	Acute	30 mg orally every 12 hours.
>12 years	Acute	40 mg orally every 12 hours.
Adults	Acute	40 mg orally every 12 hours.

	Or... 60-80 mg once daily

Steroids should not be given to people who are diabetic unless they are so bad off they'd die otherwise. Prednisone and other steroids cause their blood sugar levels to become uncontrollable. It often takes weeks or even months for their sugar to return to manageable levels. That's if the complications of high blood glucose doesn't kill them first.

A final caution regarding steroids: You shouldn't give them for more than three weeks at a time. Any longer than that, and the person won't be able to make their own cortisol - the steroid normally produced by the body - once they stop taking the pills. Their blood pressure may plummet, and they could die. Steroids, even at very high doses, are typically safe when given in short bursts of a week or two duration. Any longer than that, and the prednisone will need to be tapered down to prevent hypotension and possible shock.

Remember, it's better to give 60 mg of steroid once a day, than it is to give 30 mg twice a day. For some reason, double the dose once a day regimes, seem to cause fewer side effects.

With all these warnings, why would we even discuss the use of steroids, let alone suggest the prepper medic stock plenty in their medical kit? It's because when you need them, in certain instances, they're the only tools out there that can save lives. It would be one thing if those situations were rare, but they aren't. Severe allergic reactions, anaphylactic shock from bee stings, upper airway closure from infectious diseases. These are all disturbingly common, and for some reason, often occur when medical help is just not available.

Let's discuss the less lethal but more common conditions you can expect to see. We know these disorders will be showing up, because we've encountered them before. They're the illness relentlessly hounding the survivors of the Battle of Britain.

OTHER INFECTIONS COMMON IN A ZOMBIE APOCALYPSE

FUNGAL INFECTIONS

Another frequent infection of the shelter dwellers of WWII involves a highly contagious fungus. The moist and humid conditions, fostered by infrequent changes of clothing and the general lack of hygiene, made its contraction a sure bet.

The medical world calls these infections "Tinea"- but most of us know them as ringworm, jock itch, and athlete's foot. And while the itching alone can drive a church lady to drinking, it's the breaks in skin caused by incessant scratching that poses the real threat. Breaks here act as convenient portals of entry for bacteria; which are found in greater numbers in times of lesser hygiene.

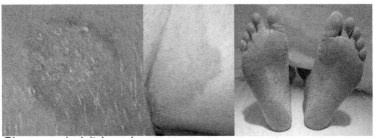

Ring worm, jock itch, and athlete's foot are all from the same fungus. Note the central clearing close-up.

Itching in the groin and feet can be un-relenting, but it is the cracking of the skin and resulting bacterial infection (cellulitis) that can be life-threatening.

Apple cider vinegar or vinegar and salt will remove ringworm. With cider vinegar, use a cotton ball to apply it onto the area being affected 3-5 times per day. It should resolve within 1 to 3 days. Vinegar and salt may also be effective, but takes up to a week to work.

Cellulitis results when entry is gained by the bacteria through breaks in the scratched up skin. Once in, they start replicating and spreading superficially, parallel to the skin.

Avoiding this means treating the fungal infection early and avoiding scratching. Antifungal creams are best if available; but apple cider vinegar or vinegar and salt will work when they're not.

Steroid creams like cortisone are to be avoided. They make the infection look as if it's receding, but once stopped, it comes back larger and itchier then before.

Cellulitis is potentially lethal. If your patient starts to exhibit this superficial spreading redness, outline the area so you can tell day-by-day if it is getting better or worse. Limit the person's activity, and keep the extremity elevated. Cellulitis took the lives of many WWII preppers. But by knowing this now, we'll be able to prevent it from taking ours.

URINARY TRACT INFECTIONS

In this chapter we'll be discussing the diagnosis and treatment of urinary tract infections. We'll show you how to check for them, and the natural remedies and conventional treatments you'll want to add to your preps.

Men rarely get bladder infections (urinary tract infections), so many of us don't appreciate how incapacitating they can be. Cleanliness can be a nightmare proposition during catastrophes. Add to that the short urethra God issued with the female bladder, and you have the first dark comedy of errors. A cruel joke of nature predisposing girls and ladies to painful infections.

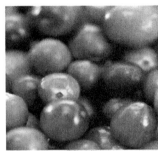
en. wikipedia.org

Cranberry juice is a proven and effective treatment for urinary tract infections. There is a chemical in the juice that prevents bacteria from adhering to the bladder wall. This helps buy the body time, so that it can expel the infection.
Forcing fluids - by drinking lots of water - can also help speed the resolution of urinary infections.

UTI SYMPTOMS

Urinary tract infections are almost always caused by bacteria. Microscopic invaders that make their way into the bladder, where they quickly set up housekeeping. Painful pelvic contractions, frequent urination, and the uncontrollable urge to suddenly go soon follow. These symptoms are sometimes accompanied by an intermittent low-grade fever. This is disastrous for preppers traveling to their Bug-Out-Locations, because walking long distances quickly becomes impossible.

WHY ARE PREPPERS SUSCEPTIBLE TO UTI'S?

In normal life you have the ability to urinate as frequently as you'd like. In concert with adequate hydration, this tends to wash out any bacteria that have made their way into your bladder. This wasn't possible for people stuck in the bomb shelters of subterranean London during WWII. Without adequate water or bathroom facilities, they quickly became dehydrated, and were forced to hold their urine for extended periods of time. Together, the combination guaranteed someone was going to get sick. Similar conditions will likely apply to modern preppers at times. Knowing this helps you anticipate the problem and implement prevention measures.

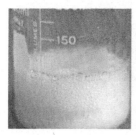 Mix 1/4 tsp of baking soda in 8oz of water and drink. Baking soda raises the pH of the irritating acidic urine produced in a UTI. This helps control symptoms until the infection resolves.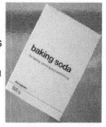

- commons.wikimedia.org

The best treatment is prevention, so stocking plenty of water in your shelter and refraining from holding your bladder is usually all that's needed. Simple steps for sure, but not always possible during an apocalypse when hygiene is its own nightmare. So preppers must be comfortable diagnosing and treating UTI's, and know how to check if the infection has spread to the kidneys.

MORE SYMPTOMS

Foul smelling, cloudy, or burning urine, combined with the physical symptoms discussed above, are all that are needed to diagnose the condition. Treatment should begin as soon as possible. Otherwise the <u>infection</u> might spread into the kidneys, *which is a potentially fatal complication.*

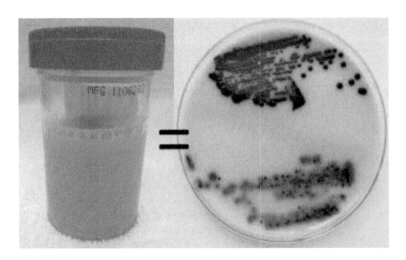

How do you tell if a bladder infection has spread to the kidneys?

A kidney infection should be suspected if a person with a UTI develops a fever that's constant or high-grade. Often the person will complain of back pain. At that point you'll want to check if the infection has extended to their kidneys. This is done by lightly tapping on the person's back directly over their lower rib cage. If they jump and recoil with sharp pain, *then the kidneys are infected!* This finding is called costovertebral angle (CVA) tenderness, and strongly suggests the person's kidneys are severely inflamed.

Pyelonephritis (Kidney Infection) & CVA Tenderness

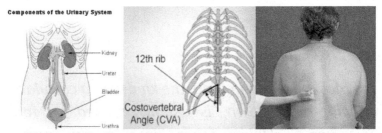

Bladder infections can extend up the ureter and into the kidney. When this happens the person may have a high fever, and severe tenderness to light tapping over the costovertebral angle on the infected side.

ONCE IN THE KIDNEYS THE INFECTION IS SERIOUS - SWITCH TO ANTIBIOTICS IMMEDIATELY.

Ideally you'll have a stockpile of people pills, but if not, fish antibiotics equivalent to Bactrim DS (<u>Sulfa</u>), or Ciprofloxin (Cipro), will generally cure the infection. If you don't get a response to treatment within the first three days, switch to another antibiotic.

The bacteria causing these infections are known to have developed drug resistance to several classes of antibiotics. So if one doesn't work, you should switch to another. In the event antibiotics aren't available, force fluids to flush the infection, improve the person's nutrition, and limit activity as much as possible. And remember: prevention, prevention, prevention!

The most violent vomiting, the kind with a calculable velocity of its own, is usually caused by food poisoning. Unlike other illnesses, this one is always preventable. But that fact alone still doesn't stop people from getting it. Let's see how it works:

POISONING FOOD

Food poisoning, or more formally foodborne illness, is any sickness you get from eating dangerous bacteria, parasites, or viruses hiding out in your food.

Usually arising from improper handling, storing, or preparation of meals; most cases are thought to be preventable by simple hand-washing.

Before the ability to routinely test for viruses, bacteria were thought to cause the majority of cases. In the field, you can often determine the type of food poisoning by its time of onset after eating. If symptoms occur rapidly, the illness is likely caused by a bacteria producing a preformed toxin. In this case the bacteria may have been killed during the cooking or canning process, but have produced and released a toxin before their death.

Staphylococcal food poisoning is a well-known example. The organism produces something called enterotoxin, which damages the intestinal wall. Within six hours the person experiences intense vomiting and often diarrhea. Severe dehydration typically doesn't occur. The toxin does its damage, then is removed by the body.

> *Food poisoning from live bacteria often cause fever, helping distinguish them from those producing preformed toxins.*

Symptoms starting 12 to 72 hours after eating point to a bacterial infection. Here the bacteria are ingested alive. Symptoms are delayed because the pathogen needs time to multiply. During replication they release a toxin, or try burrowing through the intestine and into the blood stream. Illnesses of this sort cause severe, and sometimes fatal dehydration if not treated. The bacteria need to be annihilated, or they'll continue dividing and expressing poisons or causing direct tissue damage.

Antibiotics are often needed for complete recovery. If the person has blood in their stool, they are likely infected with a species like E. coli, which directly damages the intestinal lining. Others like Cholera produce a toxin, forcing the intestines to secrete massive amounts of fluid; culminating in profound dehydration.

Viral infections make up about half of the cases in the United States. The majority are noroviruses, and like bacteria require one to three days incubation time. Most are self-limited in otherwise healthy individuals. Severe dehydration generally does not occur, the virus is destroyed quickly by the immune system.

Hepatitis A is a notable exception. It's distinguished from other viral causes by its prolonged two to six week incubation period. During that time it spreads beyond the stomach and intestines and targets the liver. People experience yellowing of the skin, a condition called jaundice. While rarely leading to chronic liver dysfunction, it's highly contagious. When people in the fast food industry are sent to the health department for their food handler's card, this is one of the illnesses being screened for.

SCOMBROID FISH POISONING

It's an illness with potentially lethal consequences - so preppers need to see it coming. Scombroid fish poisoning occurs when a fresh catch isn't kept cold enough, warming to 68 degrees Fahrenheit or above. Often it's because ice isn't available.

Since no electricity means no ice, outbreaks of this form of poisoning are common following natural disasters. Because of their northern location, this is one ailment the WWII preppers suffered from only in summer time. But for Americans, we're not going to be so lucky.

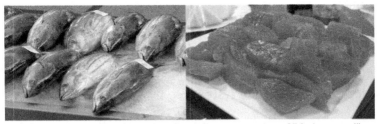

Scrombroid fish poisoning occurs from the consumption of "dark meated" fish that have been improperly refrigerated - a situation the prepper is likely to confront. A toxin is produced by bacterial action & decomposition where the naturally occurring histidine found in dark fish meat is converted into HISTAMINE - the same molecule that produces severe allergic reactions in us.

The Scombridae family of fish includes many dark meat species like tuna, albacore, mackerel, and mahi-mahi. These species contain a naturally occurring and generally harmless substance called histidine. As long as the fish are kept refrigerated this doesn't present a problem. But if the temperature rises above 68 F, the histidine turns to *histamine* - and that's bad news.

Histamine is the annoying substance our immune cells release, the one triggering an assortment of allergic reactions from hives to shock.

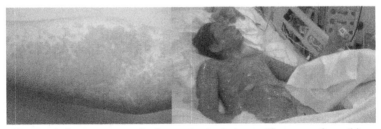

The onset of symptoms can be from minutes to hours. The range of possible effects is impressive. Flushing and facial swelling may be followed by nausea, vomiting, and severe abdominal pain. Respiratory distress and heart problems can occur, but fatalities are rare unless the person is in poor health. Untreated the condition usually resolves in 8-12 hours. Antihistamines may be of help.

> Discard fish that have been left in the sun for more than 2 hours... so you don't die!

Remember that you cannot tell if the fish is bad by its odor or appearance.   Nor is it altered by cooking or freezing after the fact.   If you must eat something - go slow.   The fish is said to have a peppery taste by those unfortunate enough to have experienced it.

FAMOUS CASES OF FOOD POISONING IN WWII WHICH MODERN PREPPERS SHOULD KNOW ABOUT

From the start, German carpet bombing proved hard on Britain's cattle population.   I sometimes wonder if cows back then dreamt of easier days ahead, when all they'd have to fear would be a random alien abduction and uterus removal.   Turns out... *Nazi's are always more terrifying than aliens.*

Regardless, the threat of protein deficiency and starvation quickly became real.   Like island nations often do, Britain turned to the sea for salvation.   Though help came at a price.

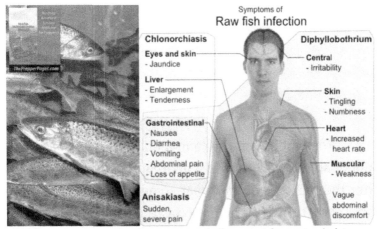

Symptoms of
Raw fish infection

Chlonorchiasis

Eyes and skin
- Jaundice

Liver
- Enlargement
- Tenderness

Gastrointestinal
- Nausea
- Diarrhea
- Vomiting
- Abdominal pain
- Loss of appetite

Anisakiasis
Sudden,
severe pain

Diphyllobothrium

Central
- Irritability

Skin
- Tingling
- Numbness

Heart
- Increased
  heart rate

Muscular
- Weakness

Vague
abdominal
discomfort

With an increased reliance on whale meat (sea steaks) in WWII, anisakis worm infections skyrocketed in the UK. Our rate will also increase, if food sources are limited to the sea.

Beef was replaced with whale meat – a meal whose identity was often disguised by parents under the simple designation "sea steak." But with this new protein source came a parasitic worm called Anisakis. No matter how well cooked, if ingested during its larval stage, could hatch into worms within the person's stomach. The infestation could range from being mild to rapidly fatal. Nausea, vomiting, and even intestinal obstruction could occur before the immune system had a chance to eliminate the infection. But that wasn't even the really dangerous part.

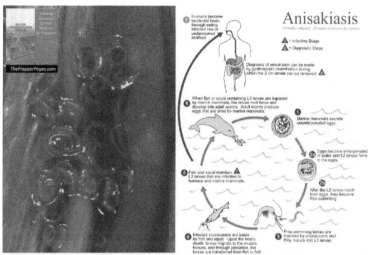

The worms are shown here in a freshly caught fish. They look like this in your stomach, & can lead to intestinal obstruction.

In a few people the worm triggered severe allergic reactions, sometimes even anaphylactic shock. Before the EpiPen became available for treating bee stings, anaphylaxis was usually fatal. Often it still is, even when occurring inside a hospital. Fortunately most allergic reactions caused by the parasite are limited to hives and mild facial swelling. You can successfully treat those with Benadryl tablets, adding prednisone if they're more severe.

WHY THIS IS IMPORTANT TO US NOW - THE SEA STEAK OF THE PACIFIC NORTHWEST

Those of us in the Pacific Northwest of the United States may find ourselves reliant on our version of sea steak – *Pacific Salmon*. Unfortunately, they too harbor the parasite. There's at least anecdotal evidence that smoking the fish may be safer than cooking it. Data suggests it might be more effective in killing the larva. For this reason we suggest smoking over cooking it whenever possible.

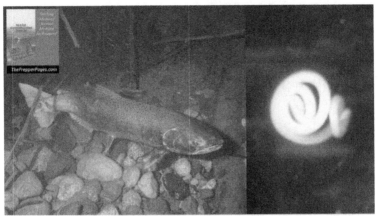

Anisakis is a parasitic worm found in pacific salmon, whales, & some other species. Typically from sushi, you can even get these when the fish has been cooked. Thousands will swim around in your stomach, and may cause anaphylactic shock.

Most of the time the infection produces symptoms limited to nausea and vomiting. But even when thoroughly cooked and killed, *Anisakis* larvae can still trigger a wide range of allergic reactions.

When you're assessing and treating a person with this complication, the trick is to gauge the degree of their allergic response. Most of the time they'll only have hives or mild asthma-like wheezing. Give them Benadryl in this instance. 25-50 mg every four hours until the hives or wheezing are gone. That will probably be the only treatment necessary. Other times more severe reactions may occur. Treatment with steroids like prednisone, or even an EpiPen may be required.   We'll discuss the route and dosage you'll use in the chapters that follow.

If the larvae hatch into adult worms, then nausea and vomiting with or without intestinal obstruction may occur. These complications are rare.   Since this parasite is not normally one of humans, it cannot survive for long in us.   *It too shall pass.*

It seems strange, but this is not the only fish preppers eat causing allergic reactions.   Another belongs to the Scombroid family, and produces its effects through a completely different mechanism.   We'll discuss it and its treatment in the upcoming chapter on asthma and pulmonary allergic responses.

The take home message is this: If a person is having an allergic reaction and you're not sure why, don't overlook fish as the possible cause.   Observe them carefully for worsening, and treat them based on the severity of their symptoms.

SECTION FIVE

WELCOME TO NATURE! DEALING WITH ENVIRONMENTAL THREATS

LIGHTNING STRIKES & MASS CASUALTIES

Did you know that there's always a lightning storm, 24 hours a day, occurring somewhere on the planet? Or that lightening does strike twice, even three times in the same place? Perhaps most surprising, is that after a strike hits people, you treat the deadest looking victims first.

Normally when confronted with multiple casualties, an explosion or airplane crash for instance, you first tend to those that might survive if treated quickly. You leave the dead - and save the "saveable." That's not the case with lightning victims. In that instance the dead are your first priority. Why you ask?

Because most of the time they'll spring back to life if you just breathe for them. The flash of blue and white current instantly overloads their nervous system, tripping the circuit breaker to their diaphragm. The self-generated electric impulses driving respiratory muscles become temporally paralyzed. So they're going to need you to breathe for them for a few minutes. Just long enough for their system to reboot.

If you perform the ventilation part of CPR, then after a few minutes they'll wake up. Completely confused at first, but in time they'll be more or less normal. The important point to remember is that once they start coughing or breathing on their own, roll them onto their side. This way if they vomit, they won't inhale what was in their stomach. *Expect they'll vomit, they just got hit by lightning.*

What about chest compressions? After a strike the heart's intrinsic rhythms will kick back in almost immediately. It's only the respiratory system takes 1-2 minutes to reset. The heart's ability to recover quickly on its own, means rarely will you need to provide chest compressions – just ventilations.

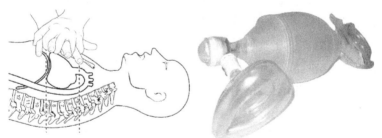

Chest compressions are not generally needed for lightning victims. If you take the mask off an ambu bag to put and use in your kit, remember it doesn't have a backflow safety valve.

HIV, Hepatitis C, and other communicable diseases are always a concern with mouth-to-mouth resuscitation. Several types of CPR masks are available to protect you. The image above shows a device called an Ambu bag. These are too big to carry around with you, but in a pinch you can detach the mask portion and use it to create a good air seal when you're breathing for someone.   The problem is it won't have a one-way valve preventing the person's secretions from coming back up and into you.

It's best to get a mask manufactured with a safety valve.   Two are shown below.   I recommend the pocket version because it saves space, and hopefully you won't be using it a lot.

Catching a disease might not be a major concern, because you'll probably be traveling with people you know well.   Besides, if you are going to die, try to do it helping someone.   I can't say for sure, but suspect that somewhere you'll get a TON of bonus points that way!

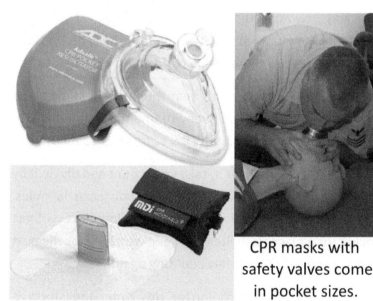

CPR masks with safety valves come in pocket sizes.

HIDING FROM LIGHTNING

When it rains it pours they say. Picture a scene where things are already going poorly, you are on your way to your bug-out-location (BOL) and tired as a dog. Now you hear thunder in the distance. "Great... that's all I need" you mutter. Resist the urge to complain to yourself, and instead *prepare to start counting.*

THE DIVIDE BY 5 & 30-30 RULES

With the next flash of lightening start counting in one second intervals. Use your favorite childhood method. Either invoke the state of Mississippi, or do the "one-one-thousand, two-one-thousand" bit. Then stop when thunder rolls. If it's within 30 seconds of the lightning, take shelter and remain there for 30 minutes (the 30-30 rule).

Sometimes you won't hear thunder but still may be in danger. Depending upon environmental conditions, you may not be able to hear it until it's as close as 15 miles.

When you do hear it, take your count and divide it by 5. This will give you the lightning's distance in miles. (Divide the count by 3 if you want it in kilometers.) Start looking for a place to shelter and keep watching for the next flash. Once you see it start counting again.

If your count was longer this time, the storm is moving away from you. You should be good. If it's shorter, be alarmed!

Let's say your first count was fifteen seconds. Your next count ten seconds. You know it's getting closer. Now calculate when it will be forming above you. Applying the divide by 5 rule (10 seconds divided by 5 = 2miles). Not so bad you might think. But remember lightning tends to strike every 2 to 3 miles. This means you're now at ground zero! Gently rest your hand on your gun or something metal, and quickly scan for shelter. If the metal starts vibrating or ringing you're really in trouble. The charge is building right above you!

Quickly order everyone to spread out and to get as low as possible. Do not shelter under an isolated tree. Make for a big thick bunch of trees instead. Do not be near the tallest structure, or somehow connected or grounded to the tallest structure.

Trees are hit by lightning even more often than water. Avoid taking refuge in shallow caves or under overhangs. The electric charge tends to splay out and reach underneath and into those areas.

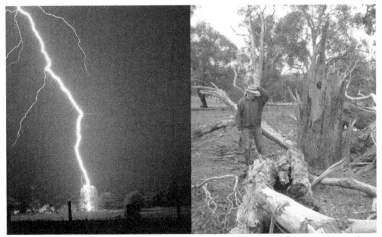

Trees hate lightning! As it strikes the tree, its heat instantly vaporizes the water within its cells, causing it to explode like popcorn. These wood projectiles can kill anyone nearby.

Most lightning injuries occur just before, or just after a storm. People either don't find shelter soon enough, or they come out too early. Strikes can occur as far as 10 miles away from the center of the storm. So it's best to remain in place for 30 minutes after the last flash.

CARBON MONOXIDE & CYANIDE - KILLER SURPRISES OF MODERN SMOKE

Stove smoke is killing more people worldwide than HIV, Malaria, and Tuberculosis (TB) combined. Deaths are currently concentrated in the third world, but it will be our problem soon. Without electricity, many people will fall back to using traditional three stone clay and wood cooking fires. While you know how to do this safely and efficiently, most people don't... and it will kill them!

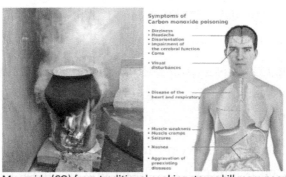

Carbon Monoxide (CO) from traditional cooking stoves kill more people than HIV! Your Pulse Oximeter will NOT help you diagnose CO poisoning!

Carbon monoxide (CO) is a colorless and odorless gas. A natural product of organic matter combustion, it's undetectable without special equipment. Sick people usually offer the first clue to its presence. Headache is experienced by most. With shortness of breath, difficulty breathing on exertion, and finally somnolence and coma all appearing as the degree of poisoning increases.

Carbon monoxide poisons people by replacing and displacing the oxygen carried by their red blood cells. The problem for both firefighters and preppers, is there's still no way of testing someone for it in the field. You'll have to go on symptoms alone. That's how it's being done currently by fire departments.

Their protocol is to assume a symptomatic firefighter, even with mild symptoms, has CO poisoning. They're automatically sent the hospital for oxygen therapy and monitoring. In years prior I'm told, they were instructed to breathe oxygen while still in the field - and shake it off. Turned out though, there was more than CO in the smoke making them sick. That changed things. I'll show you how in a minute.

If CO causes your blood oxygen concentration to decrease, why not just use your pulse oximeter to test for poisoning?

Sadly, it doesn't work for detecting carbon monoxide. The reason is interesting. Recall that the pulse oximeter measures the color of a person's blood to determine how well oxygenated it is. Bright red blood reflects good oxygenation, while dark blue indicates poor oxygen levels.

The problem is that carbon monoxide happens to turn the blood cherry red.   That's just what it does.

You can see why the pulse ox won't work now.   It see's bright red blood and thinks it's well oxygenated. While the truth is, the blood has just been dyed by the poison.

How sick will a person get?   Depends on their level of exposure.   If high enough, they'll lose consciousness, have convulsions, and become comatose.   Removing the cause or the person from the cause, along with supplemental oxygen, is about all you can do to treat it in the field.   You'll have to wait for symptoms to improve as the person's oxygenation slowly returns to normal.

Most of us know about the dangers of carbon monoxide, but few of us know about cyanide.   It's a new player in residential fires, and is causing all sorts of problems.

CYANIDE IS GOOD FOR HITLER - BUT BAD FOR PREPPERS

How do you get cyanide from burning buildings? That's a mystery that wasn't solved until recently.   It wasn't even known about until the last decade.

It started with firefighters coming into the hospital after battling residential fires, where they received the standard treatment and monitoring for CO poisoning. They had all the typical symptoms, and their blood CO levels were elevated.   But there was a lingering problem.   Even after the elevated CO levels resolved, the firefighters still had symptoms.   And that was odd.

A   bright   chemist   somewhere,   probably   an accomplished "mathlete" since high school, showed that the fiberglass insulation that's been replacing asbestos in schools and homes since the late 70s, releases cyanide when it burns!

You could almost hear Scooby's "Rut-Rho" when his findings were published.   Yep, the EPA had replaced asbestos with cyanide!

With that, the mystery of the sick firefighters was solved.   Rapid test and treatment kits made their way into emergency rooms throughout the country.   Still the problem remains: how to you test for it in the field?

Answer is, you can't.   Neither CO or cyanide blood levels can be processed outside a hospital setting.   Since both poisonings produce the same symptoms, ER physicians now routinely monitor for both.

The irony is probably not lost on you.   The WWII preppers of WWII couldn't get cyanide poisoning from fires, only Hitler did.   An end result of the fires he lit.

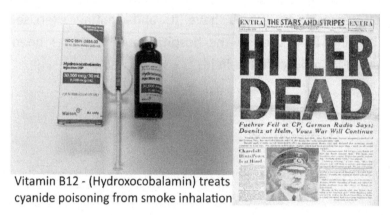

Vitamin B12 - (Hydroxocobalamin) treats cyanide poisoning from smoke inhalation

Nowadays, it's preppers most at risk.   A consequence of our government protecting us.   I'm told this is called progress.   *And I revel in its majesty!*

Recent findings show particle board also releases cyanide during combustion. Residential homes are literally stuffed with fiberglass insulation encased by particle board. So when they catch fire...

How do you know if someone has this?

One of the few unique physical signs cyanide poisoning produces, is an almond scent on the person's breath. However, only 50% of people can smell almonds in the first place. It's a genetic mutation that's swept through the world.

If you or the people you're taking care of have been in or around burning buildings, it's best to assume a headache, bluish discoloration of the skin, and shortness of breath are the consequences of both these toxins. Treat by removing the person from the environment, oxygen supplementation if you have it, and limiting exercise. Vitamin B12 is used in the hospital, but has never been tested for efficacy in the field.

Let's turn our attention to Pandemics - Dealing with the Zombie Virus!

SECTION SIX

PANDEMIC SURVIVAL SECRETS FOR ZOMBIE PREPPERS

DEALING WITH PANDEMICS

Could things get so bad you'd be forced to take care of a deathly ill loved one at home? Maybe someone infected with Ebola, or one of its terrifying friends? People across our nation are concerned there might come a time when hospitals exceed their capacity, and they'll be turned away. They're right to be concerned. But what if you couldn't even get to help if it were available? What would you do?

For decades we'd hoped this scenario would be so incredibly remote it wouldn't need to be addressed. But many of us aren't so sure anymore. SARS in China, MERS in the sand box, and Ebola... that one caught us with our pants down. The great state of Texas, one of my favorite places for sure, but even those cowboys got bitch slapped. They didn't see it coming, none of us did... save Nebraska apparently. Thank God their nurses survived. What a mess. The point being, since 1976 there have been 25 outbreaks of Ebola. In each the virus never washed onto our shores. But this time it did... *and that's changed everything.*

It might not be Ebola that causes the next American epidemic. Our last occurred in 1918 with an Influenza outbreak. It killed millions. Some speculate we're due again. Considering epidemics tend to occur every 100 years or so... *their math seems right!*

Whether or not it ever happens isn't so important. But being prepared for it is. Whether it's from SARS, a new Influenza mutant from hell, or even Ebola. This section of our zombie survival guide applies to almost all diseases with the capacity to reach pandemic levels. We use Ebola as an example, because the fundamental principles apply to all.

Nearly all of the Personal Protective Equipment images have come from the University of Nebraska Medical Center's Heroes Training Program. We highly encourage you to do two things to prepare. Sign into their site and look around. They have free downloadable posters on how to deal with chemical, biological, and radioactive contamination.

The second advice we'd offer, is to find an EMT or nurse, who can help teach you how to put in and manage an intravenous line. We've included YouTube videos on the subject, but sometimes it's helpful to be shown by someone who's done it before. Learning is faster that way. Retired military medics provide another excellent resource.

Now, let's see what we are up against.

WHAT ARE VIRUSES, AND WHY AREN'T THEY KILLED WITH ANTIBIOTICS?

Science still isn't sure why viruses exist.   Shocking to many, they're aren't even alive!   Because of this they can't be killed - *only inhibited or destroyed.*

Common to all viruses are three components: a digital code reading some sequence of A-T-C-G in various lengths and strand types, enzymes that help them replicate once in a host cell, and a protective shell called a capsid.

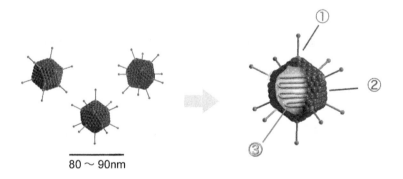

80 ~ 90nm

The virus lifecycle is pretty much the same for all, regardless of its species.   They enter your body through some type of portal - skin, respiratory system, or mucus membranes - then search for specific types of cells they can gain entry to.

Shown below is one of the viruses causing hepatitis. On its capsid – the shell in which its genetic material and replicating enzymes are contained – are receptors that brush up against the surface of your cells once inside your body.

These receptors begin feeling around for a special attachment point.   Some of our cells are displaying complementary shaped receptors on their membranes. When the correct combination is found, the two function like a lock and key.   Your cell, believing it has attached to some nutrient or material it needs, sucks the viral particle inside.   A form of molecular trickery has just taken place, and the cell won't live to make the mistake a second time.

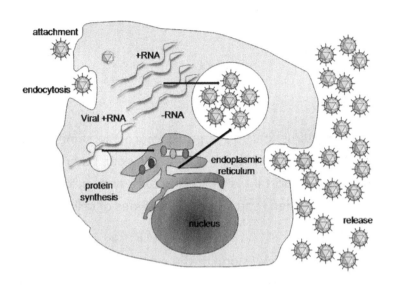

Not all viruses can gain entry into all cells.   Most can only make it into certain types, like those found in respiratory or intestinal tissues for instance.   A few have keys for nervous system cells.   Others for blood vessels or more exotic locations.   This is why certain viruses produce only certain effects.   The rabies virus for instance, can't gain entry into your nasal mucosa, but it can invade through your nerves.   Influenza invades respiratory tissue, but generally not the skin or brain.

Once in your body, some will produce strange effects by gaining access to the cells of your immune system. There they can cause the system to over secrete substances that are normally helpful in battling an infection.   In the case of HIV, the virus gains access and hides within the cells of the immune system. But in Ebola, it causes the immune system to overproduce helpful substances, which then become toxic as they reach extremely high concentrations.

After being pulled inside, the capsid falls apart. Its genetic material and enzymes then head for the nucleus, your cell's replication center. Here it hijacks the cellular machinery you normally use for replacing your own worn out tissues.

The virus cannot replicate on its own. And it's at this step the pathogen will use the enzymes it has dragged along to jump start your machinery. Using its own genetic material as a template, the process continues at rapid clip. By the time it's finished, millions of copies have been made. Not only of its genetic material and replication enzymes, but also of the proteins required for constructing its capsid.

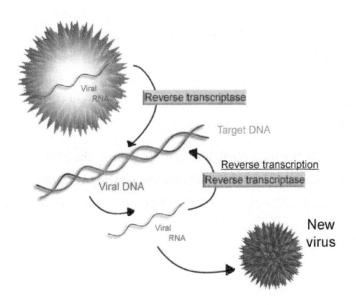

Most antiviral medications work by inhibiting the enzyme making viral replication possible. But this class of antimicrobials is still in its infancy. I'm sure you've heard of Acyclovir and AZT. These HIV medications work by tying up the viral enzymes and halting the cycle. Sadly, for Ebola, there are none yet approved for this. It seems every virus has a slightly different enzyme, and so requires a slightly different enzyme inhibitor. Designing one for each of the thousands causing human disease has proved troublesome.

Having replicated its genetic material, which can be made of either RNA or DNA, the viral enzymes and materials start pairing off. Once together they begin encasing themselves in capsids. Often these capsids are made of just two proteins. Complementary building blocks designed to intertwine and lock into place. The virus manufactures these at the same time it does its DNA or RNA. Like interlocking Lego's, they construct predictable geometric shapes.

As the viral particles come together, they hit a sort of critical biomass, and the membrane of the host cell they've invaded is split open, releasing them into the environment.

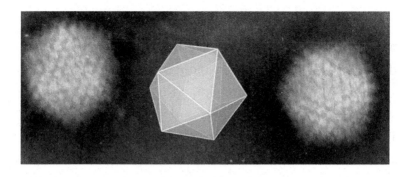

Ebola, and some other viral infections spread by contact with secretions, use a slightly different coating technique. Instead of building a capsid made entirely of protein building blocks they've manufactured, they'll use the membrane of the cell they're breaking through to cover themselves. These pathogens are called enveloped viruses. And their soft fatty-like covering leaves them much more vulnerable to soap, bleach, and other disinfectants than those geometrically shaped.

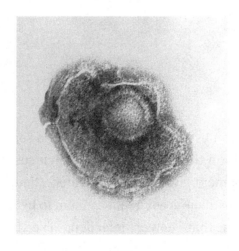

This is an image of the virus responsible for chicken pox. Notice it's an enveloped virus, and easier to transmit than Ebola. Not all enveloped viruses are equally susceptible to the environment. HIV for instance, is very susceptible, and on a countertop doesn't survive for long. That's why it must be transmitted from one person's secretions into another person's secretions to be infectious. Contrast that to a virus with a protein capsid, like those causing the common cold. Those can survive on door handles and other surfaces for extended periods.

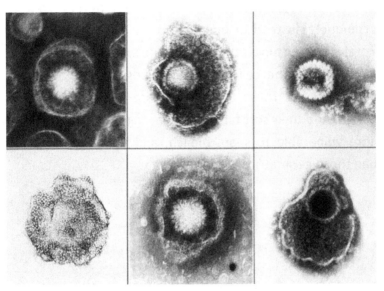

Sometimes a combination of protein capsid and host membrane form the covering, making their susceptibility to the environment variable. Other times different membranes with different qualities seem to be playing a roll. The point is that newer infections like Ebola, which

Americans have little experience treating, might behave in unusual ways. The terms of how they might be transmitted in new environments, and the contact precautions that are needed to protect people, aren't always clear. At least they didn't seem to be in Texas.

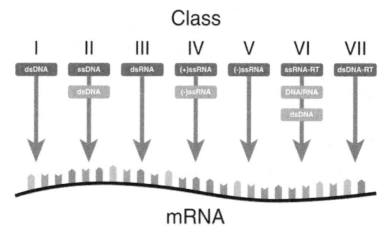

Class V: (–) ss RNA viruses (– strand or antisense) RNA (e.g. Filoviruses "Ebola").

Viruses are classified into one of seven groups depending upon their shape, and the structure of their genetic material. Ebola belongs to Group V ((-) ss RNA). A family called Filoviridae. Filoviruses are filament-like viruses, and they're brutal because many of them cause viral hemorrhagic fever – a condition where people bleed internally. The Genus and Species that's found its way to our shores is Ebolavirus Zaire - *and it too is unusual!*

AIRMAIL - EBOLA ZAIRE

Currently there are two outbreaks of Ebola. One in Western Africa, which is caused by the Zaire strain and began in Guinea in December of 2013, and another in the Democratic Republic of Congo. That outbreak began in August of 2014. In being caused by a different strain, it seems unrelated to the current Zaire outbreak in West Africa.

Our current problem began in West Africa with the Zaire strain, and is unprecedented in many ways. It's the first time occurring in West Africa. The first time in more than one country simultaneously, and the first time appearing in capital cities.

Oh... and it's the first time Ebola has appeared in the United States. That's the big one. It's also the first time it's been transmitted to Americans within our boarders. And from this point forward, we're guaranteed it won't be the last.

A recent article in *Science* suggests the virus has emerged from a strain last seen in 2004. Other peer-reviewed journals suggest its mutation rate is quite high for a virus. But we're getting ahead of ourselves. What we need to know now, is how did all of this get started?

The story begins in 1976, around the same time the World Health Organization (WHO) was about to announce that smallpox had finally been eradicated.   Since then Ebola outbreaks have been occurring sporadically, mostly in rural parts of Central Africa.   One of the reasons Ebola has become so feared, is that these outbreaks seem to come out of nowhere.   When they do, they'll kill a bunch of people - then vanish.   No one ever certain of what just happened. Let alone where the infection went to hide.   Or in what host it was finding its safe harbor.

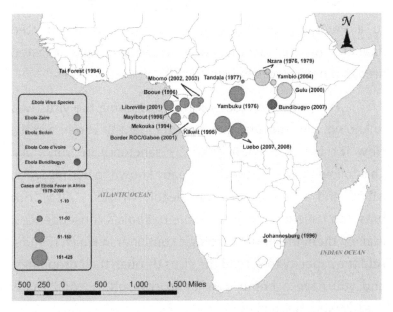

Until now, it's been this unpredictable pattern, combined with a 90% mortality rate, which has been most worrisome.   But this time... *something else changed.*

Until recently the areas hit were chiefly rural, and Ebola simply couldn't find enough hosts to muster a full-fledged pandemic. Instead it would run its course and do its damage, then disappear. Years would go by without a single case being reported. This hit and run pattern continued until the summer of 2013. When one day, in the West African heat, the virus reached an evolutionary turning point that changed everything.

In years prior the cause could always be traced back to a single person having been exposed to an infected animal. An event nearly always occurring in rural forested areas; remote places housing small nameless villages.

For years the reservoir host harboring the virus was unknown, and speculation about its identity varied widely. Now it's believed Ebola finds its sanctuary in fruit bats. This follows, because they're already known to harbor SARS, MERS, and a number of other deadly viruses. Also, fruit bats don't seem to be susceptible to Ebola's consequences, making them the perfect biologic container in which to hide. Add the capacity to spread the virus through their droppings, and you have a bomb destine to cork off. And that's exactly what happened.

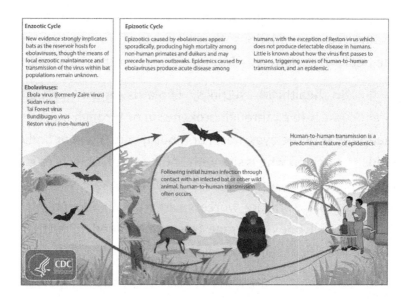

Enzootic Cycle

New evidence strongly implicates bats as the reservoir hosts for ebolaviruses, though the means of local enzootic maintainance and transmission of the virus within bat populations remain unknown.

Ebolaviruses:
Ebola virus (formerly Zaire virus)
Sudan virus
Tai Forest virus
Bundibugyo virus
Reston virus (non-human)

Epizootic Cycle

Epizootics caused by ebolaviruses appear sporadically, producing high mortality among non-human primates and duikers and may precede human outbreaks. Epidemics caused by ebolaviruses produce acute disease among humans, with the exception of Reston virus which does not produce detectable disease in humans. Little is known about how the virus first passes to humans, triggering waves of human-to-human transmission, and an epidemic.

Human-to-human transmission is a predominant feature of epidemics.

Following initial human infection through contact with an infected bat or other wild animal, human-to-human transmission often occurs.

CDC

But why now, what change in civilization made it more probable than possible?

Past outbreaks began with a person coming into contact with an infected bat, or with a primate the bat had infected. Then once into us, we'd start transmitting the infection person to person.

We tend to avoid bats in the western world. It's not so in Africa, where soups and other bat culinary dishes are considered delicacies. Monkeys aren't strangers to African palettes either. Bush meat is highly sought after in many parts of the world. Recently, it's even been finding its way into developed countries.

This point is important, because when the CDC is issuing recommendations, they're doing so for workers in the health care setting.   Not necessarily for the real world:

"In healthcare settings, Ebola is spread through direct contact (e.g., through broken skin or through mucous membranes of the eyes, nose, or mouth) with blood or body fluids of a person who is sick with Ebola or with objects (e.g., needles, syringes) that have been contaminated with the virus. For all healthcare workers caring for Ebola patients, PPE with full body coverage is recommended to further reduce the risk of self-contamination."

Source: http://www.cdc.gov/vhf/ebola/hcp/procedures-for-ppe.html

Human to human transmission is said to require direct contact with body fluids including blood, saliva, urine, feces, semen and breast milk.   It can remain in feces and semen for extended periods of time.   Even if a person has contracted the infection, then recovered.   In such cases Ebola has been found in semen as long as three months after the person has fully recovered.   In feces, it's unknown just how long it can remain viable.   No one has looked into that as far as I know.

But this is only half the story.   You can also contract the virus through certain medical surfaces called fomites. Medical instruments, stethoscopes, gloves and discarded medical waste are all examples.   Transmission from fomites is thought to require a break in the skin, but can also occur through your nasal or oral mucosa.   While intact skin offers some protection, mucosal surfaces like the mouth and eyes provide none.

No doubt you've seen the CDCs highly publicized information on how Ebola *is not transmitted*:

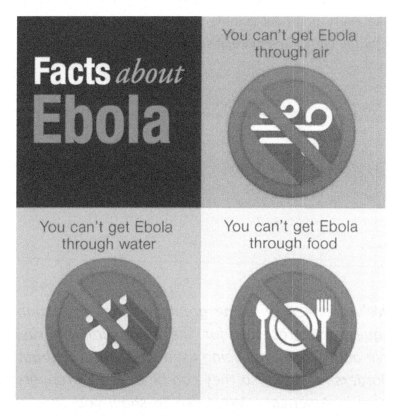

Facts *about*
Ebola

You can't get Ebola through air

You can't get Ebola through water

You can't get Ebola through food

You can only get Ebola from touching bodily fluids of a person who is sick with or has died from Ebola, or from exposure to contaminated objects, such as needles. **Ebola poses no significant risk in the United States.**

But remember, the CDC is basing these "facts" on their experience in healthcare settings. Ebola doesn't live there, it just comes to visit sometimes, leaving some of us still wondering about the possibility of it being airborne. Like every potential zombie virus it's best to assume it's airborne until you definite it's not!

We've cooked up some great personal protection equipment protocols for the next zombie virus. We adapted what's being used by Doctors Without Borders in Africa, so they can be used by preppers here in America. We'd like to show you exactly what you're going to need to survive the zombie apocalypse next!

PPE FOR AIRBORNE ZOMBIE VIRUSES

Working under the assumption Ebola virus could not be transmitted through intact skin, the CDC's initial recommendations included protective measures which still left skin of the neck and face exposed.   Then two nurses caring for the first patient unexpectedly contracted the illness, and the CDC's precautionary measures fell into question.   After a series of inexcusable blunders, their guidelines were modified – but just a little.

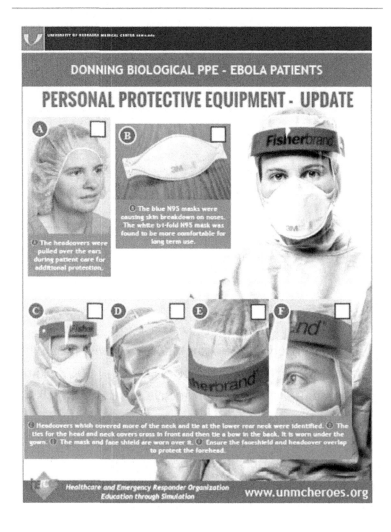

Yet the question remains for many Americans: Can you get this infection through the air?

Outside of health care facilities where "aerosolizing procedures" are being performed, the CDC contends it's impossible. They tell us Ebola cannot be transmitted through respiratory droplets suspended in the air. Even from a symptomatic person. So why is the American public still not drinking the Kool-Aid?

First, the CDC has never been able to explain how the two nurses got sick. And so for a weary public not willing to risk their lives on government guidance, an airborne transmission route remains a possibility. Animal experiments seem to support their conclusion:

- Several animal studies showing transmission without contact (Dalgard et al. 1992, Jaax et al. 1995, Johnson et al. 1995)
- An outbreak in DCR resulted in 5/19 infections in people who visited an Ebola patient but did not have contact (Roels et al. JID. 1999; 179.1)

Second, during a previous outbreak of Ebola in the Democratic Republic of the Congo in 1999, infections occurring in nineteen people were traced back to their origin. In all cases the infection had occurred after visiting a person infected - and symptomatic - with the virus. But five of those nineteen hadn't had any direct contact with the sick person, yet still caught the disease. This suggests an airborne route of infection may have been to blame.

Another anomaly is that the CDC continues to recommend only masks and face shields for health care workers, but requires respirators be used by lab personnel. This is confusing, because it's the hospital, and not the lab, presenting the uncontrollable environment. All sorts of unpredictable things happen in a hospital. That's why we watch dramas based and filmed inside them. What if a TV drama was based on a single technician working in a lab? Watching that performance would be painful!

There seems to be a lot of uncertainty around the actual mode of transmission, and this with a pathogen that has up to a 90% fatality rate. Yet the CDC concedes the possibility of airborne transmission only when health care professionals are performing "aerosolizing procedures." For instance, bronchoscopy (looking into someone's lungs with a scope) or intubation (putting a breathing tube in for mechanical ventilation). This also includes lab workers who are spinning blood in centrifuges, as that too, in theory, can generate an aerosol.

Other than those instances, it's droplet precautions only. Meaning, all you need is a surgical mask, surgical hat, and a visor to keep secretions from getting in your mouth and eyes. Oh... but also cover your skin... but you really don't have to. This is the insanity that comes with government bureaucracy – and it will kill a few people before it's all over.

Saliva and tears probably also carry some risk for the following reason: fragments of the virus have been detected in sweat, but a whole or functional virus has never been isolated from it. Because of this, the possibility of transmission by perspiration, tears, and saliva should be assumed until sufficient evidence to the contrary emerges. Preferably from studies conducted outside of Africa.

Finally, unless you're eating monkey meat or bat soup, the CDC says the illness cannot be transmitted through food or water.   Human feces, disposed of through municipal sewer system, are thought to be inactivated by the process used.   However, the CDC has not commented on individual septic systems.   In Africa, the "trench system" is typically used, and there it's obviously created problems.

The point is when a pandemic rolls ashore here, immediately adopting the highest level of personal protection you have - is the very best move.   Likely you won't even know which bug it is.   Remember illness breeds illness, so when people are sick from one, they are more likely catch and spread a second. Because it's going to be a bad scene, our advice is to be prepared to stay isolated for as long as possible!

WHEN IS A PERSON WITH A ZOMBIE VIRUS CONTAGIOUS?

Each incubation and viral shedding period is different depending upon the pathogen.   Even then there is often a great deal of variability to a single bug.

For example, the incubation period for Ebola is usually 4-10 days after exposure.   Though it can range from 2-21 days, and is why exposed people in America are being quarantined for 3 weeks.   *But people are only thought to be contagious when they are symptomatic*, because that's the only time they're actively shedding the virus.

Viral shedding is a phenomenon that occurs after an infection has taken hold in your body.   As viral particles break out of the cells they've replicated in, they're released into your secretions, and you begin sharing them unwittingly with the rest of the world.

For diseases like Influenza, you can shed the virus 24 to 48 hours before you first have symptoms.   With Ebola, the timing works out in such a way that you're physically ill at the moment you first begin shedding.   In a way, this is a lucky break.   Because you know you're not likely to get sick unless you're around an ill person. But with Ebola, what proof is there of this actually being true? How do we know people without symptoms aren't shedding the virus? How would you even test for that in Africa? It would be impossible. You'd have to have a way of knowing who was going to get sick before they do, then follow them around and check all their secretions until they became ill.

Instead, this information is being extrapolated from animal models, and making assumptions based on those might be dangerous. Think of the fruit bat for instance. He's a mammal, and he's clearly not behaving like other animal models. He doesn't even get sick, yet he still spreads the virus everywhere.

I recommend playing it safe, and error on treating it as if it were transmitted like influenza.

Since 1976 the mortality rates of Ebola outbreaks have been ranging from 30-90%. Currently, in the West African outbreak, fatalities are hovering at about 55%. No estimates of mortality rates in North America are available, mostly because we have a great deal more control over the processes Ebola uses to kill us. We have had only nine confirmed Ebola cases in the United States in the last 20 years. One of those nine died, giving us a fatality rate of 12.5%. But the small sample size and varied circumstances cannot be applied to what we might expect during an epidemic.

The main processes causing death from an Ebola infection are dehydration and hypovolemic shock. The person's blood pressure drops so low their organs cannot be perfused with blood and oxygen. These conditions are more easily treated and controlled here, than they are in Africa. Our ability to keep sick people well hydrated with intravenous (IV) fluids, and control their low blood pressure with medications, drops the risk of hypovolemic shock and fatal hemorrhage to a much lower level.

Since 1976, it's become clear that the more viral particles that make it into someone, the more ill and potentially fatal their disease will be. This absolute number is called "the infecting dose." Simply put, the larger the infecting dose of Ebola, the more destructive their disease.

This illustrates another reason personal protective equipment is so important. The two nurses who became ill while taking care the patient in Texas, both wore masks, gowns, and gloves. It's reasonable to assume their disease was less severe, at least in part, because their protective equipment limited the number of infecting organisms at the time of their exposure.

THE STAGES OF ZOMBIE VIRUSES

The progression of the infection to any specific virus is predictable.   For example, with Ebola, you come down with a flu like illness 7-9 days after exposure.   But not until day ten will you know if it's the flu or something worse.   (Of course with Ebola you will see changes in the eyes discussed earlier.)   Almost all viral illnesses start out with flu-like symptoms, then declare themselves suddenly as being either routine or fatal.   In the case of Ebola, on day ten you'll either start getting better, or progress on and experience a sudden high fever and vomiting – sometimes mixed with blood.   Day eleven is marked by bleeding from the nose, mouth, and gastrointestinal system.   Day twelve is usually the last.   The person loses consciousness and soon dies from massive internal bleeding.   Death from hypovolemic shock typically occurs as a consequence of multisystem organ failure.

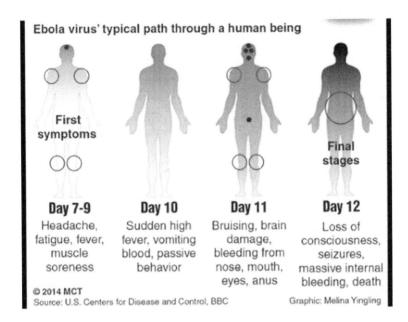

Ebola virus' typical path through a human being

Day 7-9	Day 10	Day 11	Day 12
Headache, fatigue, fever, muscle soreness	Sudden high fever, vomiting blood, passive behavior	Bruising, brain damage, bleeding from nose, mouth, eyes, anus	Loss of consciousness, seizures, massive internal bleeding, death

© 2014 MCT
Source: U.S. Centers for Disease and Control, BBC   Graphic: Melina Yingling

People that survive have fever for 5-9 days, then start to improve on day ten. Complete recovery takes weeks. In that time they'll have weakness, achy muscles and joints, headaches, and even hair loss.

How is the virus able to do this?

Ebola induces something called a cytokine storm. Cytokines are chemical messengers produced by the immune system. Traveling out to all areas of the body, they contact other immune cells and encourage them to converge on the site of infection. You've felt the effects of cytokines before. They produce the feverish, achy, and tired feeling accompanying many common colds and flus.

Cytokines, along with other molecules, also induce fever. The increased body heat speeds up enzymatic reactions the immune system depends upon, and forces the pathogen to deal with a warmer environment than it's comfortable in. Normally this response is helpful and necessary. It's also the reason many doctors don't like to treat fevers with aspirin or ibuprofen unless they're dangerously high.

With Ebola though, the production and release of these chemical helpers spins out of control. The high concentration of messengers becomes toxic, and causes massive damage to the blood vessels and organs they supply.

This is where vascular leakage and fluid loss begin. By attacking endothelial cells lining the blood vessels, cytokines cause them to start seeping plasma and proteins into tissues everywhere. Shortly afterward, microscopic clots begin to form throughout your body. These clots are quickly dissolved, but every time this cycle occurs – which is hundreds of thousands of times a minute – more of the cells necessary for clotting are used up. These non-replaceable cells called platelets, can no longer stop spontaneous bleeding that might be occurring elsewhere in the body.

The blood thins to the point you begin bleeding from your mouth, nose and intestines. Known as Disseminated Intravascular Coagulation (DIC), the process is quickly lethal. And the person dies from the low blood pressure accompanying massive internal bleeding.

PERSONAL PROTECTIVE EQUIPMENT (PPE)

We've adapted the following information is from <u>The University of Nebraska Medical Center Heroes Training Center.</u>   This is probably the best source of information we've run across.   We strongly encourage you to register at their website.   Many of the images we are about to show are courtesy of them.   Ebola is not their only concern.   At their site you can learn what equipment and procedures you'll need for dealing with chemical, biological, radiation, and decontamination threats.

In the next few chapters we'll be discussing the equipment you'll need to take care of a seriously ill person at home.   God forbid it comes to that.   The difficulty with the first protocol we'll be discussing, is that it requires you to have access to an endless supply of gloves, face shields, surgical gowns and so on.

In Africa, doctors and nurses are forced to re-use most of their equipment.   That's why you'll see pictures of them dunking their gloves, boots, goggles, overalls and other equipment in chlorine solution, then drying that equipment in the sun.   We're going to show you both systems of PPE management, American and African.   We'll be starting with that used in North America, and we'll refer to it as "The

American protocol." Use it when you have unlimited supplies.

As for the PPE management used in Africa, we'll be referring to it as "The Zaire protocol." In both cases you'll need all rubber surgical clogs, or all rubber boots. The American protocol uses clogs covered by disposable boot covers. The Zaire protocol uses rubber boots with no covering.

Shoes & Footwear

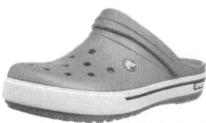 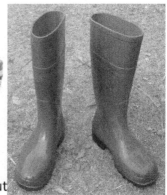

Use all rubber clogs and boots so you can soak them in bleach. Wear clogs if you're using boot covers. Use boots if you've run out

MASKS & RESPIRATORS

N95 masks come in many different shapes and sizes. Shown below are a few of them.

Some models of different masks available

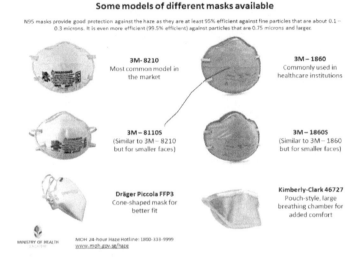

N95 masks provide good protection against the haze as they are at least 95% efficient against fine particles that are about 0.1 – 0.3 microns. It is even more efficient (99.5% efficient) against particles that are 0.75 microns and larger.

3M- 8210
Most common model in the market

3M – 1860
Commonly used in healthcare institutions

3M – 8110S
(Similar to 3M – 8210 but for smaller faces)

3M – 1860S
(Similar to 3M – 1860 but for smaller faces)

Dräger Piccola FFP3
Cone-shaped mask for better fit

Kimberly-Clark 46727
Pouch-style, large breathing chamber for added comfort

MINISTRY OF HEALTH   MOH 24-hour Haze Hotline: 1800-333-9999
www.moh.gov.sg/haze

Different N95 mask offer different levels of comfort & fit.

These are the two most commonly used:

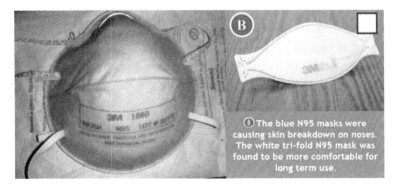

Ⓑ The blue N95 masks were causing skin breakdown on noses. The white tri-fold N95 mask was found to be more comfortable for long term use.

DISINFECTANTS, CAVIWIPES, CAVICIDE AND 0.5-1% CHLORINE SOLUTION

What's best to use for disinfecting surfaces?   Cost and efficacy have to be balanced, particularly when supplies of Purell and CaviCide are likely to be limited if an epidemic takes hold.

My advice would be to use CaviCide in high risk areas, and chlorine bleach elsewhere.   But it probably doesn't matter.   Both are effective against Ebola.

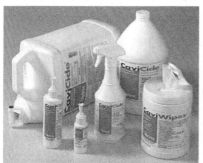 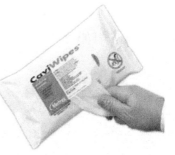

The Cadillac of disinfectants, CaviWipes & CaviCide come in many forms, but are expensive & can't be used on skin.

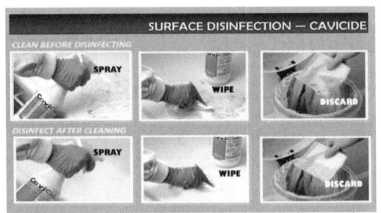

Disinfect surfaces in two stages: The first is cleaning the surface with the disinfectant, the second for disinfecting.

Regular Clorox bleach, and many of its generic equivalents, come in a standard 5% concentration. Remember to check the label, because some are as weak as 1%, while others are a stronger 10%. To make a chlorine bleach solution, pour ½ cup of undiluted bleach into 3 ½ cups of clean water. Dry the instruments before storing them. For larger batches, pour 1 ½ cups of liquid chlorine bleach into 1 gallon of water (1 part bleach per 9 parts water).

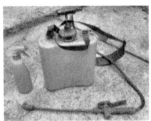 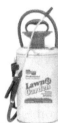

If you're going to use 0.5% bleach solution, use a metal tank with little rubber. Bleach turns rubber into a glue like goo.

COLLECTING PPE ITEMS - THE AMERICAN PROTOCOL

Two nurses caring for the first Ebola patient became ill, but no one knows how.   In response, the CDC replaced the hair cap with a full head and neck surgical cap (2).   Now, only the skin directly around the eyes should be visible. And it's to be covered with a drop down surgical face shield. This must be a shield that uses a head band, not a surgical mask with a built in plastic visor (3).   The entire head wrap visor combination should look like this:

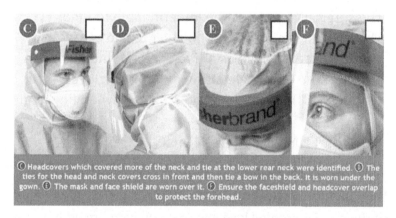

C Headcovers which covered more of the neck and tie at the lower rear neck were identified. D The ties for the head and neck covers cross in front and then tie a bow in the back. It is worn under the gown. E The mask and face shield are worn over it. F Ensure the faceshield and headcover overlap to protect the forehead.

An N95 mask, like the one shown above, should be used for patients with Ebola.   For other diseases, you can use a regular surgical mask, providing the virus you're dealing with isn't airborne.

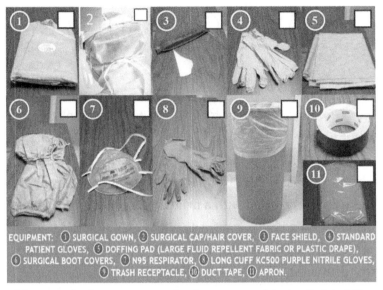

EQUIPMENT: ① SURGICAL GOWN, ② SURGICAL CAP/HAIR COVER, ③ FACE SHIELD, ④ STANDARD PATIENT GLOVES, ⑤ DOFFING PAD (LARGE FLUID REPELLENT FABRIC OR PLASTIC DRAPE), ⑥ SURGICAL BOOT COVERS, ⑦ N95 RESPIRATOR, ⑧ LONG CUFF KC500 PURPLE NITRILE GLOVES, ⑨ TRASH RECEPTACLE, ⑩ DUCT TAPE, ⑪ APRON.

The surgical gown must be impermeable to fluids (1). The surgical cap must cover all hair & skin of face & neck (2). 2 sets of gloves are needed: (4) Inexpensive vinyl & more expensive nitrile or latex (8) gloves. After placing in a biohazard bag, burn all of it when finished.

PUTTING ON (DONNING) YOUR PPE

Begin by taking off your clothing and all jewelry. Then put on scrubs or some other type of disposable clothing. Something lose and that you won't mind burning later - if you have too.

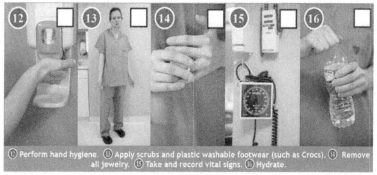

⑫ Perform hand hygiene. ⑬ Apply scrubs and plastic washable footwear (such as Crocs). ⑭ Remove all jewelry. ⑮ Take and record vital signs. ⑯ Hydrate.

Before donning your PPE, Purell your hands & remove rings. You don't have to take your vital signs, but you must drink water. The PPE is very, very hot. You'll loose fluids quickly when you have it all of it on, and you might be in it for longer than you planned.

After hydrating, put on your surgical clogs, and then slide your boot covers over them. Tie the covers up as shown in the picture. Next, put on your impermeable surgical gown. Tie the inside, and then the outside paper strings.

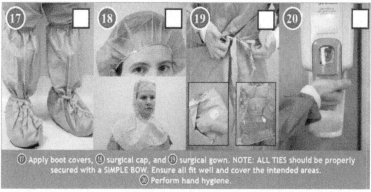

⑰ Apply boot covers, ⑱ surgical cap, and ⑲ surgical gown. NOTE: ALL TIES should be properly secured with a SIMPLE BOW. Ensure all fit well and cover the intended areas. ⑳ Perform hand hygiene.

Wear all rubber surgical clogs, not tennis shoes. Wear scrubs or clothes you can burn if needed. Put boot, not shoe covers on. Don't wear a cap (18). Use the head/neck one shown below it.

Now put on your head / neck covering. After you've tied it securely, you can put on your N95 mask.

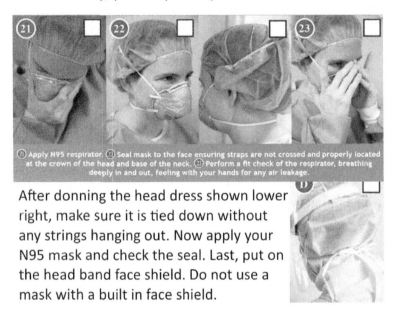

After donning the head dress shown lower right, make sure it is tied down without any strings hanging out. Now apply your N95 mask and check the seal. Last, put on the head band face shield. Do not use a mask with a built in face shield.

After your face shield is on, wash your hands with Purell again, and put on your inexpensive nitrile gloves. Pull the gown's cuffs over the nitrile or latex gloves.

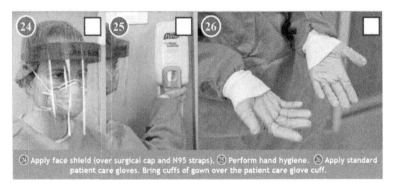

Next apply your second set of gloves, the purple nitrile or yellowish latex gloves, over the top. Make sure you order nitrile or latex gloves with long cuffs (KC500). Otherwise, if they are short cuffed like the first pair you put on, you won't be able to duct tape them to the gown correctly.

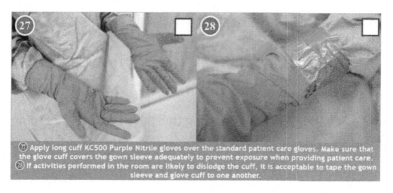

Apply long cuff KC500 Purple Nitrile gloves over the standard patient care gloves. Make sure that the glove cuff covers the gown sleeve adequately to prevent exposure when providing patient care. If activities performed in the room are likely to dislodge the cuff, it is acceptable to tape the gown sleeve and glove cuff to one another.

After your long cuffed gloves are on, and have been pulled up over the sleeves of the gown, duct tape them into position as shown.

Remember to fold the duct tape back on itself, and make a tab when you do this, so you can peel if off easily when you're finished!

Please watch and download this video. Then make your own copy for review later, as it's easy to forget the details.

University of Nebraska Medical Center Heroes Ebola Donning Video

https://www.youtube.com/watch?v=yAIjqBcqnP4&feature=youtu.be

Removing (Doffing) PPE – The American Protocol

Even if you plan on using the Zaire protocol, learning the American protocol is still necessary. It shows you the principles of donning and doffing you'll need to apply to your reusable PPE.

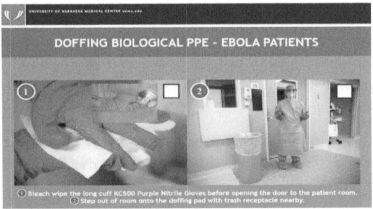

This is one of the most important steps, & often overlooked. Door handles can be lethal if not cleaned. Keep bleach wipes in the room!

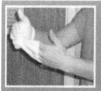

Remove exam gloves using glove-in-glove technique. Dispose of gloves onto the doffing pad with the discarded suit and hood.

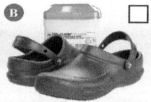

Please see the American Red Cross "how to" on glove removal

Ⓑ Before staff members step from the doffing pad to the floor, the top and bottom of each shoe is bleach wiped.

Once you receive your supplies, practice the glove-in-glove technique until it's second nature. It's this step, I think, where the Texas nurses may have contaminated themselves. That's not because they didn't know what they were doing, but because the technique is difficult.

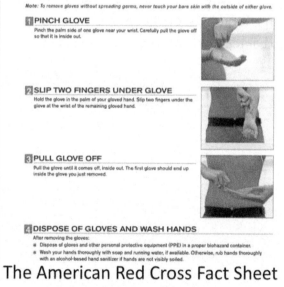

The American Red Cross Fact Sheet
www.in.gov/isdh/files/BBP

Notice the tab the nurse created with the duct tape. Doing that makes it so much easier to remove.

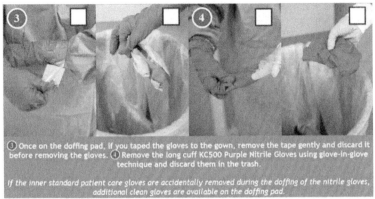

③ Once on the doffing pad, if you taped the gloves to the gown, remove the tape gently and discard it before removing the gloves. ④ Remove the long cuff KC500 Purple Nitrile Gloves using glove-in-glove technique and discard them in the trash.

If the inner standard patient care gloves are accidentally removed during the doffing of the nitrile gloves, additional clean gloves are available on the doffing pad.

Use the glove-in-glove technique every time you take them off. Practice by dipping them in chalk, then see if you have on you.

Regardless of how you've decided to tie your gown, you mustn't leave any of the strings hanging. They can come into contact with infected fluids much too easily!

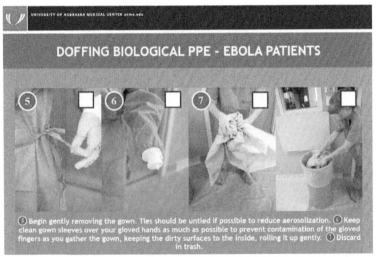

UNIVERSITY OF NEBRASKA MEDICAL CENTER unmc.edu

DOFFING BIOLOGICAL PPE - EBOLA PATIENTS

⑤ Begin gently removing the gown. Ties should be untied if possible to reduce aerosolization. ⑥ Keep clean gown sleeves over your gloved hands as much as possible to prevent contamination of the gloved fingers as you gather the gown, keeping the dirty surfaces to the inside, rolling it up gently. ⑦ Discard in trash.

There are 2 ties, one outside (shown) & one inside. You may not want to tie the inside, in case your under-gloves are contaminated.

Rolling the boot covers down in sections is safest. That way only the interior surface of the cover is exposed. This too, takes some practice. It's best to practice the technique before you actually have to use it!

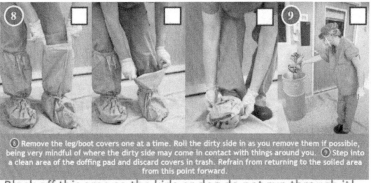

⑧ Remove the leg/boot covers one at a time. Roll the dirty side in as you remove them if possible, being very mindful of where the dirty side may come in contact with things around you. ⑨ Step into a clean area of the doffing pad and discard covers in trash. Refrain from returning to the soiled area from this point forward.

Block off this area so the kids or dog do not run through it! Make sure you can get to your bio-trash bag from off the pad

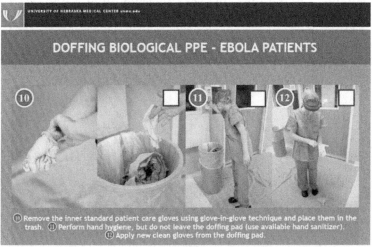

UNIVERSITY OF NEBRASKA MEDICAL CENTER unmc.edu

DOFFING BIOLOGICAL PPE - EBOLA PATIENTS

⑩ Remove the inner standard patient care gloves using glove-in-glove technique and place them in the trash. ⑪ Perform hand hygiene, but do not leave the doffing pad (use available hand sanitizer). ⑫ Apply new clean gloves from the doffing pad.

You'll want to set up your doffing pad outside, before donning your PPE. Place your Biobag, Purell, & gloves on pad.

Block off all areas. If your dog brushes up against an infected surface, it's gave over!

The picture below illustrates your next step: removing the face shield.   Try to use this instead of a mask with a built in shield.   That two-in-one combination offers far less protection.

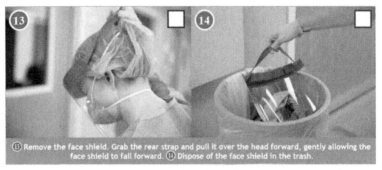

⑬ Remove the face shield. Grab the rear strap and pull it over the head forward, gently allowing the face shield to fall forward. ⑭ Dispose of the face shield in the trash.

The order of removal is important to remember!

Try to avoid these hair bonnets, and use head covers instead.   Sometimes this isn't possible, and it's better to use this type of cap, than no cap at all.

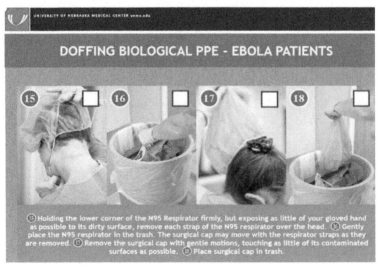

DOFFING BIOLOGICAL PPE - EBOLA PATIENTS

⑮ Holding the lower corner of the N95 Respirator firmly, but exposing as little of your gloved hand as possible to its dirty surface, remove each strap of the N95 respirator over the head. ⑯ Gently place the N95 respirator in the trash. The surgical cap may move with the respirator straps as they are removed. ⑰ Remove the surgical cap with gentle motions, touching as little of its contaminated surfaces as possible. ⑱ Place surgical cap in trash.

Take off mask, then your head covering!

Last, roll your floor pad up into a ball, touching the outside or undersurface only.

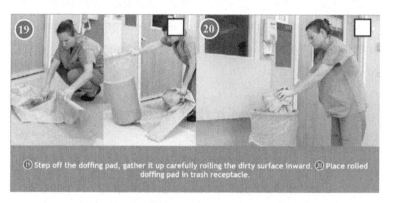

⑲ Step off the doffing pad, gather it up carefully rolling the dirty surface inward. ⑳ Place rolled doffing pad in trash receptacle.

Here is their video, please review it and make a personal copy for yourself later.

University of Nebraska Medical Center Ebola PPE doffing instructional video

http://youtu.be/D95r0dEETsI

THE ZAIRE PROTOCOL (WE ARE GOING TO TWEAK IT FOR ZOMBIE PREPPERS

In total, the reusable items for the Zaire Protocol cost about $90. The goggles, tunic, apron, trousers, and protective gloves are sanitized and reused, whereas the other wearable items are used once, and then placed in your bio-bag and burned.

Items Needed for the Zaire Protocol

- **Rubber surgical apron**
- **Surgical trousers and tunic**
- **Wraparound protective goggles**
- **Anti-fog spray (for goggles)**
- **Gloves**
- **Rubber boots**
- **Hood**
- **Cape**
- **Respirator mask/face protector**

The short two minute video below is included here to show you what is being used in Africa.

What to wear in an Ebola outbreak zone

http://youtu.be/yUm90Tiyz4M

THE PROTOCOL

When putting on equipment, workers should adjust for comfort and should not adjust in the treatment center because of the risk of exposure and contamination.

Preparation

1. Wash hands.
2. Put on coverall or gown, tying at back of the neck and waist.
3. Secure facemask or respirator and make sure it fits snuggly around nose bridge, face and below chin.
4. Place face shield or goggles over face and/or eyes.
5. Surgical cap ties at the back of the head.
6. Boots or shoe covers are positioned and worn underneath the gown. Some workers wear two layers.
7. Apron ties at the back and loops to the front.
8. First pair of gloves is worn under the cuffs of the coverall or gown.
9. Second pair of gloves is worn over the top of the coverall or gown, in some cases, gloves are taped shut by a buddy.
10. Each person puts on their own gear, but each worker has a buddy. The buddy spot-checks for tears in equipment or open areas of skin that could become contaminated.

In the treatment area

11. When treating patients, workers should not touch their own faces, should limit the number of surfaces they touch, change gloves if heavily contaminated and wash their gloved hands often.
12. Depending on the organization or the availability of gloves, workers must either change the outer layer of gloves when moving from patient to patient or wash gloved hands with soap and water.

SOURCE: Centers for Disease Control and Prevention.

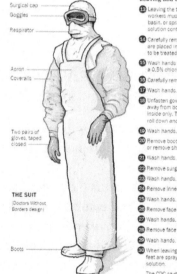

Surgical cap
Goggles
Respirator
Apron
Coveralls
Two pairs of gloves, taped closed
THE SUIT (Doctors Without Borders design)
Boots

Leaving and undressing

13. Leaving the treatment facility, workers must step into a chlorine basin, or spray or wash with a water solution containing 0.5% chlorine.
14. Carefully remove outer gloves, which are placed in a biohazard container to be treated and incinerated.
15. Wash hands with soap and water or a 0.5% chlorine solution.
16. Carefully remove apron.
17. Wash hands.
18. Unfasten gown ties and push gown away from body by touching the inside only. Turn gown inside out and roll down and over boots.
19. Wash hands.
20. Remove boots with a boot remover, or remove shoe covers.
21. Wash hands.
22. Remove surgical cap.
23. Wash hands.
24. Remove inner layer of gloves.
25. Wash hands.
26. Remove face shield or goggles.
27. Wash hands.
28. Remove face mask or respirator.
29. Wash hands.
30. When leaving the containment area, feet are sprayed with bleach solution.

The CDC cautions workers not to bypass any of these steps.

There are two important points regarding the Zaire protocol. First, removal of the PPE requires a buddy who's there to spray bleach and spot any break in protocol. The second, is to notice that they are washing their gloved hands - every step - after they've removed their outer protective pair.

For this, they're using a water cooler filled with bleach solution, and set up on a table in a makeshift decontamination facility (please see video). While doing this, their standing on a patch of ground they've dug a pit in, and filled with rocks. That way the water will filter down below the level of their boots, and they can fill it in later with dirt. Step-by-step, it breaks down as follows:

DECONTAMINATION & DOFFING STEPS

After leaving the treatment facility, or your home quarantine room, step into a chlorine basin, or spray or wash with a water solution containing 0.5% chlorine.

1. Then remove outer gloves, and place them in you bio-bag and container to be treated and incinerated.
2. Wash your hands (still wearing your under-gloves) with soap and water or a 0.5% chlorine solution.
3. Carefully remove your apron.
4. Then wash hands your gloved hands again.
5. Unfasten the gown ties carefully, and push it away from your body by touching the inside only. Turn the gown inside out and roll down and over your boots.
6. Wash your gloved hands again.

7. Remove your boots with a boot remover, or remove shoe covers.
8. Wash gloved hands again.
9. Remove your surgical cap.
10. Wash your still gloved hands again.
11. Remove the inner layer of gloves.
12. Wash hands.
13. DWB does not do this, but I recommend putting on another pair of gloves, like you do with the American protocol, at this stage. Remember how you put clean gloves on your floor pad outside the room for use while doffing? I strongly suggest you add that step here.
14. Remove face shield or goggles.
15. Wash hands (gloved).
16. Remove face mask or respirator.
17. Wash gloved hands.
18. Take off gloves for good.
19. Wash ungloved hands.
20. When leaving the containment area, your feet are sprayed with bleach solution.

SOURCE: Centers for Disease Control and Prevention.

The video below shows how they are doing this in Africa. Start at 19:22 minutes. Watch what they do, then make it fit your needs at home.

http://youtu.be/6lb6WblKyRE?t=19m22s

The best way - by far - to reduce the mortality of Ebola, Zombie, or any other deadly virus, is to aggressively hydrate them. This is the single most important thing you can do to save your loved ones. So... let's learn how to do that next!

ACCESSING & TREATING DEHYDRATION

It's clear now. The best way to treat Ebola is by keeping the victim well hydrated. If they're dehydrated, then fluid replacement is mandatory. This applies to other zombie viruses, but probably not to the degree it does with Ebola.

Ebola does its damage by creating a dehydration that's so profound in a person, their blood pressure drops and their internal organs die from lack of oxygen. This is called multisystem organ failure, and it's often accompanied by a disorder called DIC, where random blood clots form and then dissolve, in all the person's blood vessels. This quickly uses up all of the blood clotting cells called platelets. And the person begins bleeding everywhere, until their blood pressure drops to critical.

The first rule of treating children and adults suffering from dehydration is the most important. It says you should always rehydrate the person with oral fluids when you can. The gastrointestinal system does a much better job of absorbing water and electrolytes, and distributing them to the rest of the body, than is possible with intravenous (I.V.) rehydration.

Pedialyte is a favorite of mothers who are trying to keep their little ones hydrated during a stomach virus. But it's expensive. Gatorade is very similar in electrolyte concentration, and far less expensive. So many of us recommend using it instead of Pedialyte. Oral rehydration solutions (ORS) work best when given in small amounts often, instead of in larger amounts hourly. This also helps prevent nausea and vomiting, both common in Ebola and other deadly infections.

If you have access to water, the best way to orally rehydrate someone is by using powdered electrolyte replacement packets. They take up little room, are inexpensive, and basically last on a shelf forever.

You'll want to avoid putting in an I.V. at home, unless you really have to. Even if you have to give anti-nausea medications like Phenergan - so they can continue to take electrolyte solution orally – it's better than using an I.V. That being said, when you need one, you need one. We'll show you how to put one in shortly. For now, let's review the signs and symptoms of dehydration, and how to access its severity.

Symptoms of dehydration very from person to person, but several are common to everyone. Age also plays a role in what symptoms the person has. Dehydration symptoms in a child will not be the same as those in a teenager, adult, or elderly person.

To access the level of dehydration in a child, look at their general condition. The more severe their dehydration, the more lethargic, restless, or irritable they'll be.   Look to see if their eyes are sunken, or if they're able to make tears.   Look in their mouth for saliva.

Next pinch up their skin over the abdomen.   Do this like you would with the ruff on the back of a dog or cat's neck.   In a well hydrated person, the skin will drop right back down after you release it.   The more dehydrated they are, the longer it takes to fall back into position.   If it takes longer than 2 seconds, they are dehydrated.   For children, if their tongue is dry they are at least 3% dehydrated, if they're crying but not able to make tears, they're at least 5% dehydrated.

Classifying Dehydration

Remember that the more dehydrated you are, the less urine you'll be making.   If a person is adequately hydrated, they will be making at least 20 ml of urine an hour.

Dehydration is often divided into three groups. Group A includes those with no dehydration.   Their sick, but their volume loss is less than 3-6%.   Just keep them hydrated through their illness with ORS, and replace any fluids they lose.

For children up to 2 years of age, give them 50-100 ml after each episode of vomiting or diarrhea they have. Add this to the "maintenance fluids" you're making them drink so they won't become dehydrated.   If they are older than two, then give 100-200 ml after each stool.

If a child or adult vomits the ORS, wait 10 minutes, then have them sip it more slowly - and give less.   In both children and adults who are not continually vomiting, anytime they want more solution, give it to them.

Group B is divided into mild and moderate dehydration.   The mild from indicates they have lost 3-6% of their fluid volume.   Their pulse will be normal, or only slightly elevated (60-100 BPM in adults).   They will have decreased urine output, and the person will be thirsty.   To calculate how much fluid replacement they will need, multiply 50 ml by their weight in kilograms (kg).   In mild dehydration, the skin will tent for 2 seconds or less.

Moderate dehydration comes from having lost 7-10% of their body fluid.   These people will have an elevated heart rate >100 (tachycardia).   They may be either irritable or lethargic, will have no tear production, and be making little or no urine.   Their oral membranes and tongue will be dry.   Mild tenting of the skin, often for greater than 2 seconds, will occur when you pull up on their abdominal skin.

Treating Group B Dehydration in Kids	Give the amounts below in the first 4 hours			
Age	Up to 4 months	4-12 months	12-24 months	2-5 years old
Weight	< 5 kg	6-10 kg	10-12 kg	2-5 years old
In ml	200-400	400-700	700-900	900-1400

Click Here to See Enlarged Table

To calculate how much fluid you'll have to replace, multiply 80 ml by their weight in kilograms.

Group C is made of those with severe dehydration. They have lost > 11 – 15% of their fluid volume, and will be in the first stage of shock. Their pulse will be rapid and weak. Their blood pressure will be very low. They won't be making any urine. They'll have cold and mottled skin.

If you are comfortable with putting in and managing an I.V. line, put it in at the moderate stage of dehydration. Try not to wait until the dehydration is severe... *if you can help it.*

SECTION SEVEN
TREATING LUNG CONDITIONS PREPPERS CAN EXPECT TO GET

Lung Conditions Plaguing Preppers

Our lung section is packed with important information and easily learned skills. You'll be able to start applying both immediately. We're going to teach you what a doctor is thinking and looking for, when evaluating infections, coughing, shortness of breath and other breathing problems. We're going to show you how to do what they do, so you can save your friends and family. *Even your daughter's boyfriend if you want!*

Lung infections and chest trauma were the biggest killers of those caught in The Battle of Britain. But that part was predictable. Infection and injury have always been the closest friends war has ever had. Inseparable since the first hairless apes started throwing rocks at one another, the three have grown up like siblings. And their tight relationship has shown no signs of weakening over ages of human conflict.

Locked in half-step behind the anger and fog of war, you can expect a visit from the trio to our shores soon.

EXAMINING LUNGS & THUMPING MELONS

Of all the conditions we looked into, bronchitis and pneumonia were two of the most serious and frequent the WWII preppers faced.   Other than trauma, these lower respiratory tract infections conferred the greatest risk to life. Bronchitis usually isn't fatal, but it often leads to pneumonia – which ended up killing many.

Smoke from smoldering ruins, musty closed in spaces, and a frequent and close proximity to one another did many in.   It was a killer combination they never seemed capable of escaping.   An inevitable consequence of bomb shelter life, it snuffed out the young and old without remorse.   It was insanity.

The good news is with inexpensive equipment and a few exam skills, you can easily make sense of any respiratory problem.   Best of all, understanding these conditions is not difficult… it's all mechanical.   There's no magic or formal training needed.   You can learn it in a remarkably short time!

Bronchi, Bronchial Tree, and Lungs

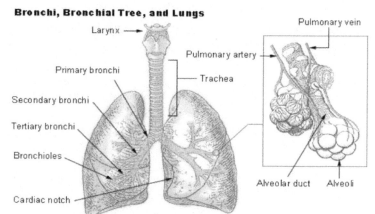

Larynx →
Pulmonary vein
Pulmonary artery
Primary bronchi
Trachea
Secondary bronchi
Tertiary bronchi
Bronchioles
Cardiac notch
Alveolar duct   Alveoli

There are three major places lung conditions can reside. The air tubes (bronchi & bronchioles) which have hairs called cillia that clear mucus upward. The lung & chest wall lining (pleura). And the air sacs called alveoli.

THE FOUR STEPS TO FIGURING IT ALL OUT

Start by thinking about the structure of the respiratory system as it's shown in the picture above. There's a throat, trachea, bronchi, lungs, air sacs, two outer lung linings, and a potential space in-between the lung and the rib cage. That's it. If something's wrong with a person's respiratory system, it will be in one of these places.

Next, have the person tell you about the symptoms they're having. Then listen to the lungs with your stethoscope and percuss their chest wall. Finally, use your pulse oximeter and peak flow meter to take readings. Let's go over each of these steps separately.

377

After reviewing the anatomy in your mind, and asking them to tell you about their symptoms, examine their throat and lungs. Using your stethoscope, begin by listening for "extra lung sounds."

What Are Extra Lung Sounds?

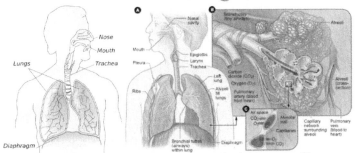

Anything obstructing or constricting the airways will cause unique lung sounds to be heard when the person breaths. Each area, from mouth to lung base, has a signature sound!

HOW AND WHERE DO YOU LISTEN WITH YOUR STETHOSCOPE?

Begin by placing it on the person's back; after they've removed their shirt. Ask them to take deep breaths through their mouth. If they breathe through their nose, you often won't be able to hear the subtle sounds revealing what type of illness they have.

Remember to listen all the way through the person's complete inhalation and exhalation. Many problems in the lung can only be heard, or are heard best, during the end phases of respiration. Try to force yourself to wheeze right now, and you'll see what I mean.

Heathy lungs produce soft and gentle breath sounds which you can barely hear.   Any change from that indicates something's wrong.   Listen to your own lungs with your stethoscope to see what normal lungs sound like.   If you don't have a stethoscope yet, put your ear to someone's chest and listen.

Start on the anterior chest wall, move to the sides, and then work your way down the back from areas 1-4 as shown.

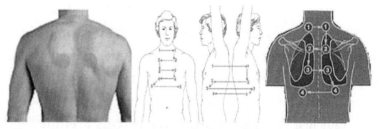

The purpose of listening over the lung fields with your stethoscope is to see if you can hear adventitious or "extra" breath sounds. Auscultating over the anterior or lateral chest can be helpful, but the area between the shoulder blade and spine (circled areas 1-4 in the far right figure) is most productive. This is also where you "tap" or percuss.

As you get farther down, you'll notice the soft breath sounds you heard clearly up in area 1 & 2, will get more and more difficult to hear.   This is because the lungs are ending, and the person's diaphragm is beginning.

On the right side in the lower level marked by the circled 4, you'll won't hear anything.   That's because the liver lives here... and it's solid.   Knowing where it's at is helpful because you can use it as a reference point.   For instance, when we start percussing - tapping over the lung fields - to see if the person has pneumonia, it will sound just like it does over the liver, if pneumonia is present.   Let me clarify:

As we'll see, pneumonia is a collection of puss that localizes in large segments of the lung.   When you listen to segments of lung that have pneumonia, they sound just the same as when you're listening over the liver.   Likewise, when you percuss over lung segments that have pneumonia, it sounds just the same as when you percuss over the liver. In both instances they sound dull.

But sometimes you'll forget what dull is supposed to sound like.   In that instance, you can go back and tap over the liver, which always sounds dull.   Then use that sound for comparison!   If the person has dullness where there are usually soft air sounds, then pneumonia may be present. We'll go into this more soon.

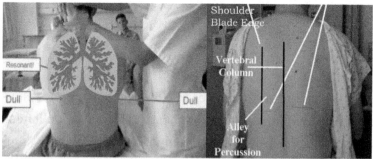

The purpose of listening to lung sounds & percussing for dullness is to determine if the person has simple bronchitis, or if they have a more serious condition called pneumonia. These examinations will also help tell you if the person is getting better or worse. Notice that percussion is done in an "alley" between the spine & shoulder blade.

Chest percussion is done with the middle finger of one hand, tapping on top of the middle finger of the other hand, using a snapping wrist action. The stationary hand is placed firmly on the back between the inside edge of the shoulder blade and the spine.

Chest Percussion

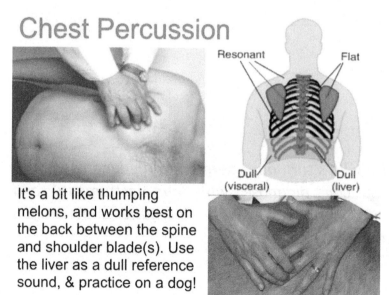

It's a bit like thumping melons, and works best on the back between the spine and shoulder blade(s). Use the liver as a dull reference sound, & practice on a dog!

A dull sound indicates the presence of puss or fluid collections within the lungs or chest. Normally you'll hear a resonant drum-like sound when percussing over lung fields, indicating these air-containing structures are healthy. The technique was initially used to distinguish between empty and full barrels of whiskey and wine, but works similarly with human lungs.

Now let's turn our attention to the lung conditions we can diagnose with our instruments and examination techniques. It is easier and more fun than you'd think!

ASTHMA, ANAPHYLAXIS, CARBON MONOXIDE & BRONCHITIS

The large airways supplying the lungs begin centrally, then splay outward towards the periphery like the branches of a tree. Becoming smaller in diameter and more numerous as they make their way to the air sacs at their terminal ends. These air sacs are called alveoli, and are where oxygen and carbon dioxide exchange with the bloodstream takes place.

Lining the airways are small hair like structures called cilia. These microscopic heroes of the war on germs, are continually clearing microbes entrapped within the mucus that's lining the airways. Beating in an upward direction, they bring particulate matter, viruses, bacteria and other inhaled debris trapped within the mucus, up to the throat where it can be cleared and swallowed.

Yes, this is what's happening when you clear your throat!

This highly coordinated system starts to fail when smoke and other inhaled toxins paralyze the cilia, thereby preventing removal of these contaminated secretions. The consequences can range from frequent infections, to life-threatening allergic and asthmatic like reactions.

ASTHMA

Asthma is a condition characterized by wheezing and shortness of breath. Using your stethoscope, you'll hear wheezing mixed in with normal soft breath sounds.

Better described as "reactive airway disease," asthma is a condition where air passages suddenly spasm and constrict in response to an allergen or irritant.

Asthmatics also have a dry cough at times, one that sounds very unique. If you have a friend that has a child with asthma, ask them to call you next time they have an attack. Then listen to their cough. Once you've heard it, you'll not mistake if for anything else. Then listen to the kid's lungs so you can hear what wheezing sounds like. Sometimes it sounds more like "honking" than wheezing. That's really the best way of learning to recognize the disorder.

WHAT CAUSES ASTHMA?

While cigarette smoke has long been known to paralyze the respiratory cilia, smoke from the fires inevitable to war and catastrophes is just as toxic.

Both asthma attacks and bronchitis frequently follow in the wake of such scenes. Having no control, there's little you can do for someone but treat these conditions as they take hold of a person.

Typically you'll treat the wheezing part of asthma with an inhaler. If it was caused by an allergic reaction, you also treat the allergy with Benadryl when mild, prednisone when moderate to severe, and with an EpiPen if severe.

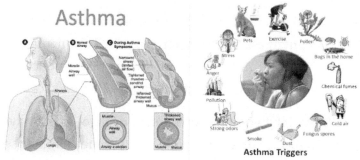

Asthma results from sudden constriction of the airways. Turbulent airflow in this condition causes wheezing or "squeaks" at the end of the persons exhale (so loud, often you don't even need a stethoscope) But remember "all that wheezes is not asthma." Severe allergic reactions & anaphylaxis also constrict the airways & cause wheezing!

Degrees of bronchoconstriction can range wildly, from mild with minimal wheezing, to a feeling of impending suffocation and the certainty of death. Attacks of this severity often impede air movement so completely, the person can no longer even produce a wheeze. This is bad! *You must inject the person immediately with an EpiPen.* Once they're able to swallow, give them prednisone, Benadryl, and humidified oxygen if you have it.

Reactive airway disease is not exclusive to asthma. Better thought of as a reaction pattern, you'll frequently see it accompanying other lung conditions like bronchitis, pneumonia, and pulmonary edema (fluid in the air sacs).

If the inhaler didn't help much, or if you don't have one, the meter is still very useful. Take a measurement a couple of times a day to see if the person's condition is getting better or worse. Along with your pulse oximeter, it can help you decide if more aggressive treatment is necessary.

ANAPHYLAXIS & ALLERGY

Allergic reactions can range in severity from mild wheezing and puffy eyes - to anaphylactic shock. It's often said to young doctors in training: "all that wheezes is not asthma." Meaning several diseases, allergens, and toxins produce this squeaking sound.

Many lung infections, most notably bronchitis, produce some degree of airway spasm. The result is a musical whistling sound best heard on end expiration... a finding known on the street as wheezing.

HOW DO YOU TREAT BRONCHOSPASM & WHEEZING?

An EpiPen is a lifesaver in severe reactions. Benadryl tablets are helpful in less aggressive cases. Like when wheezing is minimal or absent, and hives or facial swelling are the only symptoms.

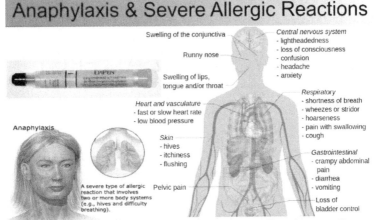

Anaphylaxis & Severe Allergic Reactions

Swelling of the conjunctiva

Runny nose

Swelling of lips, tongue and/or throat

Heart and vasculature
- fast or slow heart rate
- low blood pressure

Anaphylaxis

Skin
- hives
- itchiness
- flushing

A severe type of allergic reaction that involves two or more body systems (e.g., hives and difficulty breathing).

Pelvic pain

Central nervous system
- lightheadedness
- loss of consciousness
- confusion
- headache
- anxiety

Respiratory
- shortness of breath
- wheezes or stridor
- hoarseness
- pain with swallowing
- cough

Gastrointestinal
- crampy abdominal pain
- diarrhea
- vomiting

Loss of bladder control

Anaphylaxis is like a full-body severe allergic reaction. Often you will hear wheezing before the person's face starts to swell. Tx with Epi-pen, Prednisone & Benadryl.

Prednisone falls somewhere in-between.

Use your pulse oximeter and peak flow meter to monitor the person after you've given them Benadryl. If they're not improving after a while, or are getting worse - reach for your prednisone.

You'll need it for our next couple of chapters too. They contain some strange ailments. Illnesses I'm sure the WWII preppers would have wanted to know about. They were frequently affected by them, but these conditions were unknown to science at the time. And oddly... they're caused by a fish!

BRONCHITIS

An infection of the lower airways, bronchitis is usually caused by a virus.   From it, the WWII preppers suffered terribly.

Most often resulting from a widespread viral infection of the airways, bronchitis is the perfect setup for developing a subsequent bacterial pneumonia.   The ball gets rolling when the viral pathogen invades the cells lining the airways, sometimes all the way down to the air sacks. This leaves delicate lung tissue open to attack from bacteria. The germs all of us normally inhale from time to time. Bacterial invasion of the ravaged lung tissue results in pneumonia.

For WWII preppers, the combination of smoke and uncirculated air in the shelters proved disastrous. Triggered by particulate matter suspended in the air, bronchitis seems to be an inevitable consequence of smoldering buildings, burning tire piles, and other silliness accompanying urban chaos.

An educated guess as to virus or bacteria can help you here.   If it's bacterial, then you can club it with your favorite antibiotic. To guess, apply the rules we discussed earlier, but tweak them a little so they'll work for the respiratory system.

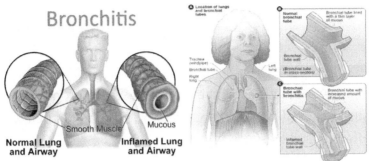

Bronchitis

Normal Lung and Airway

Inflamed Lung and Airway

Smooth Muscle

Mucous

Bronchitis is an infection of the airways and is usually caused by a virus. It results in the build up of mucus which is audible when the person breathes. This turbulent airflow produces something called rhonchi... and sometimes wheezing. Rhonchi are coarse "cruddy" or "mucusy" hacking sounds that clear or move around with coughing

The following rule of thumb can be applied for most infections of the pulmonary system – sinuses all the way to the lung lining.

Remember, viral infections tend to be carpet bombers. You'll see indiscriminant destruction of whatever cells they manage to con their way into. For example, the flu typically gives you a runny nose, sore throat, swollen eyes, cough, vomiting, and pneumonia.

Contrast this to a bacterial infection like Strep throat. Here you'll experience a sore throat; possibly a fever. Maybe some swollen neck glands. Do you see how it's sort of localized in a way? Seems bacteria usually invade one area at a time. Only after establishing a stronghold will they work their way into the sinuses, lungs, or wherever.

With bronchitis you'll often hear a wet cough, and rhonchi when listening with your stethoscope.   You might also hear wheezing.

My advice on how to best treat it would be the following: If a person has this "bacterial pattern," you're justified treating them with antibiotics right away.   If they have the widespread symptoms typical of a virus, save your antibiotics and make them comfortable.   Test to see if an inhaler will help them if they're wheezing.   Use your peak meter to see if you get a response.

I'm I doctor, so I'm obligated by years of brainwashing to repeat my parties' favorite line: "push fluids – lots of fluids."   But now I'll tell you why.   Water thins secretions better than any medicine.   Clearing mucus becomes much easier after thinning it with copious amounts of water.

This one's also reflex: "lots of fluid - *but no milk!*" Since it's a thick fluid, people think it thickens secretions. But the real reason we advise against it, is because if the infection is viral, it's probably already infected your patient's intestines.

Entering and destroying superficial cells in the lining, the virus causes a temporary lactose intolerance.   These are the cells containing lactase, the enzyme responsible for breaking down lactose in milk so that it can be absorbed. Without it they'll get diarrhea, and be adding a new layer of misery onto their current illness.

Within two weeks these damaged cells will have finished replacing themselves with functional copies, and the person will be able to return to drinking milk and eating cheese.

Now let's talk about the conditions causing water or infected fluid to fill your lungs!

FLUID & INFECTIONS IN THE LUNGS AIR SACS

Remember our discussion on melon thumping? Here's where knowing how to perform chest percussion pays off.

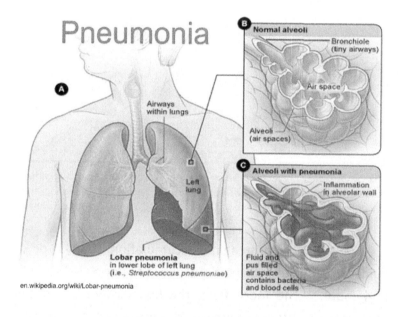

As you've probably gathered, we're working our way farther and farther down to the deepest recesses of the lung and chest cavity. Approaching our discussion this way allows us to visualize these conditions systematically, based on their location.

You can use this framework – working from the throat all the way down to the lining of lung – whenever you are trying to figure out the cause of a person breathing problem.

At this level we find ourselves at the terminal end of the airways – the air sacs.   Known as "alveoli" in medicine, this is the area where the actual exchange of carbon dioxide for oxygen in the bloodstream takes place.

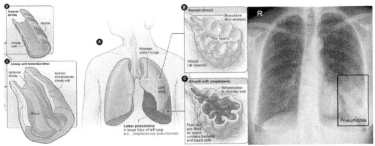

Shallow breathing prevents the lower parts of the lung from expanding with air, so mucus builds up & the air sacks collapse. Bacteria then set up shop, and the person can develop pneumonia (see far right). Rib belts can make it worse.

As you might imagine, accumulation of any type of fluid within these alveoli will impede one's ability to oxygenate.   The more fluid, the less oxygen – and the greater the shortness of breath the person will experience.

In the case of pneumonia, the fluid is generally pus. A thick mixture of fragmented bacteria, spent immune cells, and mucus with different degrees of viscosity depending upon its water content.

Tip: An expectorant is any medication of substance that thins thick secretions. Mucinex is a well know OTC expectorant, but drinking lots of water has been shown to be even more effective. It also avoids the stomach irritation that often occurs with that medication.

The mixture doesn't stay liquid for long though. It quickly consolidates like Jell-O would in a refrigerator. This semi-solid substance must be broken down by the body with enzymes, and is why it can take months for pneumonia to fully resolve.

When coughed up, the sputum of pneumonia is usually foul-smelling and may be rust or gray colored, depending upon the bacterial species responsible.

Rarely do people go from being well, straight to contracting pneumonia. Usually they'll have had another respiratory infection first. They may have even seemed to be getting better. But then suddenly they become febrile, develop a productive (sputum producing) cough, and feel short of breath.

Now we come to the melon thumping. Percuss over the lung fields, listening for dullness as you do. Areas of lung filled with pus are called "consolidations," but are not the only finding characteristic of the infection. You can also use another test, called egophony, to help tease out areas of consolidation.   <u>Click here for a one minute video.</u>

http://youtu.be/5ONKdBD8Ff8

While listening to the chest with a stethoscope, have the patient say the vowel "e" over two or three seconds "e-e-e-e."   Over normal lungs, the same "e" sound (as in "beet") will be heard with your stethoscope.   If the lung is consolidated, indicating the person has pneumonia, the "e" will take on a nasal sound and change to an "a" (as in "say").

If you're not sure of the difference, use the same trick we discussed before.   Perform egophony first over the patients lung fields until you hear "e-e-e-e," that will be your normal control spot.   Then repeat the test with your stethoscope over the liver.   It should sound like "a-a-a-a" due to the liver's tissue density.   That's your pneumonia control spot.   Now return to the lung fields to see if consolidation is present.

I find this technique more accurate and easier to perform than percussion.   Both work the same way; they point out abnormal changes in lung density indicative of pneumonia.

Let's say that you've just found an area with dullness to percussion or egophony.   Or just have someone with shortness of breath and a cough.   So now what do you do?

This is how you put it all together into a plan of action:

EVALUATING COUGHS
TREATING LUNG INFECTIONS

You are helping someone with a cough and maybe some shortness of breath.   Their cough may or may not be productive, it doesn't really matter.

The goal is to see how sick they are, so you can gauge how to treat them.   For instance, a person with bronchitis can probably travel by foot for short distances, whereas a person with pneumonia will require bed rest and close monitoring.

Start by measuring their oxygen saturation level with your pulse oximeter.   The lower the reading, the sicker they are, and the more rest they need.

Next use your meter to determine their peak expiratory flow.   Compare that reading to the chart that came with the device.   Record both your patient's pulse ox and peak flow measurements for future reference.   This will help you tell if they're getting better or worse over the days to come.

Now listen to the lungs.   Note any areas you hear rhonchi, wheezes, or other extra breath sounds somewhere in your notes.   Percuss over the lung fields and use

397

egophony to see if you can pick up any areas of consolidation.

If you cannot find consolidation, the person probably has bronchitis.   If they do have dullness, then presume they have pneumonia, or fluid from some non-infectious cause in their lungs.

Finally, refer to your initial peak flow and pulse ox readings, then give the person a few puffs from your inhaler. Recheck your readings with both instruments 5-10 minutes later.   Now compare before and after findings to predict if albuterol inhalation is likely to help them.   I should note that albuterol also comes in pill form, for use with uncooperative children.   It's easy to give to them, but has more of the hyperactive and nervous side effects than the inhaled preparation.

TREATING BRONCHITIS & PNEUMONIA

Augmenting and Cipro should both work for treating most cases of pneumonia. Sometimes an erythromycin antibiotic like Zithromax is required. This is especially true if the organism causing the infection is unique. These pathogens don't fit the typical profile for a "bacteria."

You may already be familiar with this problem – the infection they produce is called "walking pneumonia." Mycoplasma is one such organism... and it hates erythromycin type antibiotics. Though, like all organisms, has developed resistance over the years.

Further treatment may consist of albuterol inhalations; if they help increase the person's peak flow, or if they improve their symptoms of shortness of breath. Pushing fluids to thin secretions, and limiting physical exertion will also be necessary.

SHOULD BRONCHITIS EVEN BE TREATED WITH ANTIBIOTICS?

That's a tough question even for doctors. You know that bronchitis, which looks much like pneumonia without the findings of consolidation, is most often caused by a virus.

So many of us base the decision of whether or not to use antibiotics on how long the person's had bronchitis. Two weeks without improvement is where I have drawn my sandy line, though I may use them earlier if there are compelling reasons.

You'll want to avoid giving antibiotics to a person who's recently come down with bronchitis, for the sole purpose of trying to prevent it from progressing to pneumonia. In medicine we did this early on, because like most decisions we've made over the years, it seemed like a really good idea at the time. It turned out to be a mistake.

Doctors found out later, regardless of the organ system involved, giving antibiotics prophylactically actually increases the risk of getting a bacterial infection. They'll kill off the friendly bacteria living in the area. This is counterproductive, because they normally compete against the harmful ones.

Both good and bad bacteria are always locked in a struggle for resources and living space. We call this "competitive inhibition" and antibiotics can quickly tip the balance in an unfavorable direction. They can do more harm than good.

What if I've given someone antibiotics, but they don't seem to be getting better?

This happens frequently, and is frustrating for everyone involved. As for specific antibiotics, you'll probably have to try one and watch for a week or so to see if you get a response.   If you don't, and the person doesn't seem to be getting better, then switch to a different antibiotic.

There is so much antibiotic resistance out there, it's often hit and miss.   Antibiotics belonging to the penicillin, sulfa, erythromycin (Z-Pak and others), and Cipro family's seem to work best.   Seven to ten days is the typical treatment duration.

All sorts of things can cause your lungs to fill with water.   None are good, but most are treatable. We'll discuss how to save people with these conditions next!

DROWNING WITHOUT WATER - PULMONARY EDEMA & CHF

Have you ever known anyone with congestive heart failure (CHF)? It frequently follows a heart attack. The heart, having been injured and lost some of its pumping power, is unable to propel the normal volume of blood out to the periphery. As a result, pressure builds up in the lungs and fluid seeps into the air sacs. When severe, the person "drowns internally."

Because the fluid collects distal to the airways, wheezing is often minimal or absent. So how do you hear fluid? You listen for Rice Krispy's!

Rales a.k.a "Crackles"

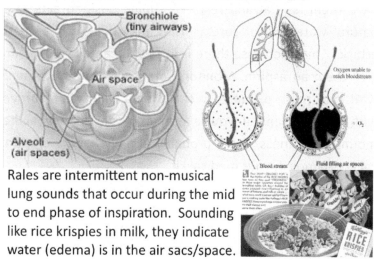

Rales are intermittent non-musical lung sounds that occur during the mid to end phase of inspiration. Sounding like rice krispies in milk, they indicate water (edema) is in the air sacs/space.

Water pills, called diuretics in medicine, can help remove the excess fluid. Fortunately though, CHF is rare in most situations you'll encounter. The exception is when it occurs from being at high-altitudes. This condition, called high-altitude pulmonary edema, causes fluid to rush in to the air sacs. Your group members may suddenly start coughing up pink frothy sputum. Good times!

Your patient's will also be short of breath, and have a low pulse ox readings. They will have crackles or rales in their lungs, and when you perform percussion, the lungs will seem dull on both sides.

Regardless of the cause, pulmonary edema is treated much the same way.

If a person has rales, and you don't have diuretics, have them lay flat and rest. A supine position acts as a natural water pill of sorts. They may have had a heart attack. In which case there is little you can do other than give them an aspirin. Monitor worsening or improvement with your pulse oximeter. The edema will likely improve with diuresis, and if you're prepared for treating acute mountain sickness, you'll probably already have a diuretic called Diamox in your medical kit.

Let's learn more about high-altitude illness and treating pulmonary edema now:

Altitude, Acute Mountain Sickness, High-Altitude Pulmonary Edema (HAPE) & Hangovers

Unexpectedly, and sometimes against your wishes, you'll find yourself being pushed back and up into mountainous areas. While these high peaks may not be part of your bug-out-plan, it's important to know how to deal with acute mountain sickness in case you find yourself there.

A recent example of this occurred in the summer of 2014. A terrorist group calling themselves I.S.I.S, cloaked in ninja costumes and running around like idiots with pirate flags, pushed the Kurdish people of Northern Iraq to hill tops within a mountainous region. It's more accurate to say they fled to elevation in effort to avoid the heavy armor of the invading force. You may remember the NATO helicopter airlifts tasked with evacuating the wounded and sick. Many individuals had been injured during combat, while others, largely women and children, were evacuated because they were suffering from altitude sickness.

These peaks were not excessive in elevation.   As such, they illustrate two important elements to this disease. First, it's random; one cannot predict who will be affected. Second, the speed of ascent seems to be related to disease severity – as well as the overall number of people effected. In other words, if you're forced to run uphill because you're being chased by tanks, expect higher rates of acute mountain sickness than if you strolled up casually.

In the United States, acute mountain sickness is experienced by 15% of people visiting a Colorado ski resort. Even higher rates are found in mountain climbers.   This probably reflects the degree of exertion inherent to the sport (see the table below).

Described best as a spectrum of disease, altitude illness reflects an incomplete response by the body in its attempt to adjust to elevation.   This spectrum can range from simple acute mountain sickness - producing symptoms similar to a hangover - to those of fluid retention in the lungs (pulmonary edema) and sometimes brain (cerebral edema). These more severe forms confer a higher mortality rate.

Acute	Mountain	Sickness		
Location	Colorado Resort Skiers	McKinley Climbers	Rainier Climbers	Flown to an Elevation

				of >14K feet
% of People Affected	15%	50%	70%	70-100%

WHAT IS ALTITUDE ILLNESS?

It's commonly believed, as elevation increases, the air's oxygen concentration decreases. In reality, the oxygen concentration stays the same. It's the barometric pressure that decreases. Known as the "partial pressure of oxygen" in medical circles, barometric pressure is the driving force of oxygen. The energy pushing it from your lungs, into your blood stream.

At 14,000 feet, this driving pressure is about half that at sea level. As a rough estimate, this means only half the normal amount of oxygen will be pushed into your blood stream. Your body must compensate.

Here's how:

Your breathing rate, or respiratory rate (RR), increases in the first few days. At the same time there is a water diuresis – a dehydration resulting from excessive urination – that serves to functionally increase the concentration of your red blood cells (RBC's) per unit of blood. Excreted with the water is a base called bicarbonate, which helps keep the blood pH neutral.

Acute mountain illness is a benign disorder that generally resolves in a day or two, due to the compensatory mechanisms of the body described above. Symptoms include one or all of the following: headache, insomnia, lethargy, loss of appetite, nausea and vomiting, and mild shortness of breath.

It's helpful to think of the disorder as if it were a hangover. Sometimes you'll just have a sort of "mental fogginess." Often the 15% or so of skiers affected never realize they have AMS. Instead, they attribute their symptoms to the alcohol typically consumed during the first few days of a of ski vacation.

Symptoms can begin at elevations as low as 8,000 feet. Sometimes even lower - as in the case of the Kurds. But symptoms increase substantially from this point, with every additional 1,000 feet ascended. For instance, at 8,000 feet, the base elevation of a typical ski resort, 15% of people suffer from AMS. But at 10,000 feet, 50% of people are affected.

To avoid this, once you've hit 8,000 feet, try to limit your ascension to 1000 feet a day. And remember the higher you go, the less altitude you should gain each day.

Elevations 12,000 feet and above may produce profound water retention in the lungs, a disease called high-altitude pulmonary edema. It may even produce cerebral edema severe enough to induce coma (high-altitude cerebral edema). Regardless, anytime you travel above

10,000 feet, expect some minor cerebral edema leading to mild lethargy and confusion.

High Altitude Illness Table HA	Acute Mountain Sickness (AMS)	High Altitude Pulmonary Edema (HAPE)	High Altitude Cerebral Edema (HACE)
Location	>8,000 feet	Usually >10,000 feet	>12,000 feet
Time	1-2 days after ascent	3-4 days (or later) after ascent	4-7 days (or later) after ascent
Symptoms	Headache (H/A), Lethargy, Sleep disturbances, Anorexia, Nausea & Vomiting	Shortness of breath at rest, Weakness, Cough, (Can progress to Pink Frothy Sputum)	Severe headache (H/A), Confusion, Hallucinations
Physical Signs	Mild increase in heart rate (HR), possible edema of extremities	Increased HR **and** Respiratory Rate (RR), Fever, Cyanosis	Ataxia (unsteady gait) and other neurological or visual signs, Retinal Hemorrhages
Treatment	Rest at same altitude or descend to sleep, Hydration, Mild analgesics, Restart ascent in 1-2 days:	Descend immediately, Oxygen if available, acetazolamide & Dexamethasone 4 mg every 6 hours, (both are unproven but	Descend immediately, dexamethasone 8 mg bolus then 4 mg every 6 hours, hyperbaric therapy if available

	prophylaxis and treatment with acetazolamid e (Diamox 250 mg 2 X day)	experientially and anecdotally effective), Hyperbaric therapy if available	
Copyright 2014	**ThePrepper-Pages.com**		

The best treatment for all forms of altitude illness is descent.   This isn't always possible.   For instance, when tanks are waiting for you at the bottom of the hill.

If you can move down a bit, try sleeping at a lower elevation than you've ascended to that day.   This is thought to help speed the acclimation process.   And that leads us to the first of two practical medicines you'll want to have in your kit for treating this condition.

Pulmonary Edema HAPE & CHF

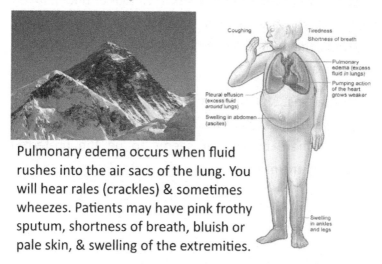

Coughing

Tiredness
Shortness of breath

Pulmonary
edema (excess
fluid in lungs)

Pumping action
of the heart
grows weaker

Pleural effusion
(excess fluid
around lungs)

Swelling in abdomen
(ascites)

Swelling
in ankles
and legs

Pulmonary edema occurs when fluid rushes into the air sacs of the lung. You will hear rales (crackles) & sometimes wheezes. Patients may have pink frothy sputum, shortness of breath, bluish or pale skin, & swelling of the extremities.

Acetazolamide, also known by its trade name Diamox, produces effects mimicking and accelerating the body's compensatory mechanisms discussed earlier. It's a diuretic that causes water loss, effectively increasing the number of oxygen carrying red cells per unit of blood.

One of the most useful aspects of this medication, is its utility as a prophylactic treatment. If you know you'll be at elevation, start taking it one to two days prior to ascent. You can even start the medication at the beginning of your climb - as might be needed if you have to flee upward unexpectedly.

Diamox tablets are scored and breakable, making it easier to customize their dosage. They are available in 125 mg and 250 mg tablets, and can be given to children as well as adults.

When used for prevention, the dosage is 5-10mg/kg/day in two divided doses.   This is continued for 48 hours.   If you are using it on someone already having symptoms, the dosage frequency doubles to 5-10 mg/kg/day in 3-4 times daily.

The last medication to discuss is the steroid dexamethasone.   Typically given in its I.V. form, we only mention it here because it seems to be the preferred treatment in the movies.

The most frequent complaint of people at altitude is a sore throat and ear pain.

We would suggest not giving steroids for altitude illness, unless you're forced to by severe shortness of breath or neurological symptoms.   Even then, it might be better to treat the person with the steroid you already have in pill form - prednisone.   You've probably already stuffed it into your kit for instances of severe allergic reactions and asthma.

One last tip about altitude.   By far the most common complaint of those at elevation is sore throat and ear ache, sometimes with a cough that resembles the signs and symptoms of bronchitis.   But these symptoms are not from an infection.   They're caused by a combination of the dry air intrinsic to elevation, and the ongoing dehydration from diuresis and water loss inherent to the acclimation process.

Ear pain results from Eustachian tube dysfunction, the same thing you may recall experiencing on your last flight. Treat these complaints by humidifying the air, perhaps by inhaling steam from water you boil, and chewing gum to help open the Eustachian tube.

We're getting to the gruesome stuff. Let's talk about the really, really dangerous things next!

CONDITIONS OF THE LUNG LINING, CHEST WALL, & POTENTIAL SPACE - PLEURISY

Between the linings of the chest wall and lung, resides a tiny amount of straw-colored fluid.   Known as pleural fluid, there's typically just enough to create a suction cup type seal.   Imagine a glass of ice water sitting on a glass table during a warm day.   If you try to pick it straight up, the suction cup action keeps the glass affixed to the table's surface.

Fluid around the lung functions in a similar manner. Between the visceral and parietal pleura - the tissue layers lining the chest wall and lung - is a small collection of fluid. One functioning like that between the glass and table. Almost magical in design, this suction-seal allows the lung to be pulled and to expand with air effortlessly as your respiratory muscles contract and travel outward during inspiration.

Anatomy of the Pleural Space

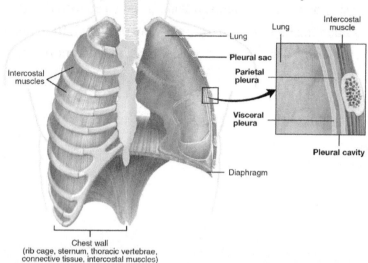

Chest wall
(rib cage, sternum, thoracic vertebrae,
connective tissue, intercostal muscles)

Two slippery surfaces cover the lung & chest wall. The lining adherent to the lung is called the visceral pleura, the one adherent to the chest wall is the parietal pleura. Between the two - blood, fluid, or air can accumulate.

PROBLEMS IN THE SPACE WITH THE SUCTION-SEAL

Here's the problem: This space can potentially fill with too much fluid, or even air. That's what's occurring with pneumothorax. Even with just a little of either, the suction cup seal is lost, and the work of breathing increases significantly. But it gets worse.

If it fills with fluid, or more commonly air, as is frequent with trauma, the pressure can build up and push the lung into the heart. You know that an air collection between the lung and chest wall is called a pneumothorax. But if enough accumulates, it will not only collapse the lung, but push the heart over to one side and prevent it from filling with blood.   This is known as a tension pneumothorax – and it's lethal.

Pleurisy, Pneumothorax & Pleural Effusion

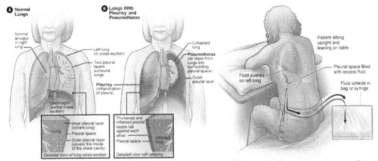

The pleura (lung lining) can become inflamed from trauma & infection - a condition called pleurisy. Both fluid & air can become trapped between the lung & the chest wall. If the collection is air, it's called pneumothorax & when percussing sounds hollow. If fluid collects, it's a pleural effusion & is dull.

HOW DO YOU TELL IF SOMEONE HAS A PLEURAL EFFUSION OR PNEUMOTHORAX?

In both instances you may no longer hear the soft sounds of air moving in and out of healthy lungs when listening with your stethoscope.   You often lose sounds altogether on the affected side.   The trapped fluid or air is collapsing the lung and pushing it towards the heart, so there's no air filling the lung to hear.   All you hear... is nothing!

So which is it?   Fluid or air?   Here's where percussion comes in.   When you percuss over a chest full of air, you're essentially tapping on a drum, and you'll hear a tympanic resonant sound.   If you get these two findings together - no moving air and tympani to percussion - then you know the person probably has a pneumothorax.

When you percuss over a chest full of fluid, you're essentially tapping on a melon or full keg of beer, and you'll hear dullness.   If you get these two finding together – no moving air and dullness to percussion – then you know the person probably has a pleural effusion.

Of the two, pleural effusions are best tolerated. They can be drained, and this will help the person breathe easier.   But that's more than you'd want to take on in the field.   It's also unlikely to cause problems with blood not being able to return to the heart.   You won't see the same consequences we talked about with tension pneumothorax.

Pleural effusions are uncommon in situations preppers are likely to face.   It's a pneumothorax and a tension pneumothorax that are the monsters under the bed. And those demons are real.

CHEST TUBES

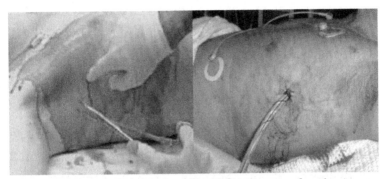

Inserting a chest tube can be difficult even for doctors. It's impractical for preppers to attempt this in the field. Performing needle decompression with an improvised I.V. catheter is a much more reasonable option. Chest tube insertion really needs to be done in a hospital.

Some survival medicine books teach the procedure for placing a chest tube, like the one shown above, for treating a person with a pneumothorax. We're really not sure why. It requires a lot of analgesia, a water seal sterile collection chamber, and a post-operative chest x-ray. None of which are typically accessible to preppers.

Years ago there was a story in the news about a person who had just been in a car accident. He was banged up a bit, but late for a flight he needed to be on. Rushing from the scene, he skipped the hospital and went directly to the airport. Boarding the plane with sore ribs and a bit of a cough, he thought he'd be okay. Within about an hour he couldn't catch his breath. He had that feeling sometimes washing over a person... he knew he was going to die. He almost did!

Fortunately, there were two physicians on board.

He'd sustained a rib fracture in the accident, and a sharp bone fragment had lacerated his lung. Air escaped and collected under pressure between his lung and chest wall. He had a pneumothorax. Short of breath and turning blue, the doctors could tell it was evolving into a tension pneumothorax. They didn't have a stethoscope, so they placed their ears against his chest wall to determine which lung collapsed.

Yes, they'd been in lecture the day the history of the stethoscope was discussed.

Without decompressing the chest - letting the air out - blood flow returning to the heart would be squeezed off in minutes. The hurried traveler would have been a goner.

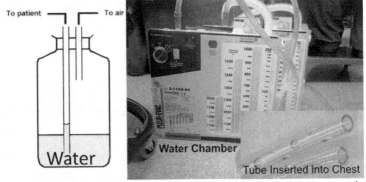

The doctors on the airplane improvised a water seal chamber using a coffee pot and some tubing they found. How they were able to insert a large bore tube like this without analgesia is a mystery to us.

With the help of a flight attendant, the doctors scavenged through the galley for a large tube, and something that would serve as a water chamber. They found a coffee pot, filled it halfway with water, and inserted tubing cut from a drop down oxygen mask into his chest. The air rushed out and the person lived.

I've was told later, for their trouble, the airline sent each of the doctors a medium-sized fruit basket.

I find that the most predictable part of the story!

What were they doing with the half-filled coffee pot? Turns out that placing the other end of the tubing - the one extending out from the person's chest - under water to create a seal is essential. It allows the built-up air exiting the chest to pass through the tube and bubble out into the water. At the same time, the water seal prevents outside air from being sucked back through the tube and into the chest.   A situation often occurring with open chest wounds and unsealed conduits.   Without a water seal, or some other way of occluding the exiting end of the tube, air will always rush back in through that conduit when the person inhales.   You'd get nowhere.

You may be wondering, if placing a chest tube is not practical for preppers, why are we discussing it? Well, the tube isn't so useful, but the principles of chest decompression are.   Particularly the parts regarding the water seal.   Somehow, you're going to have to figure out how to close of the exiting end of any tube you use to decompress the chest. That's coming up now!

NEEDLE DECOMPRESSION & ONE-WAY VALVES

Now to the really good stuff! We're going to discuss a different technique for treating pneumothorax – one you can actually use. Instead of using a chest tube, we'll be working with a large bore I.V. catheter, and something to seal it. You may not be able to fix up a water seal, but there's easy way to get the same effect. You can improvise a one-way valve!

A flutter valve, also known as a Heimlich valve, is a one-way control device used for preventing air from travelling backward into the chest.

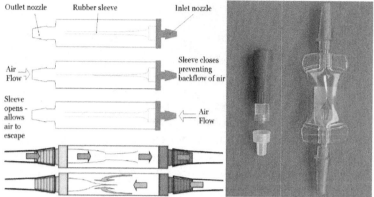

Outlet nozzle   Rubber sleeve   Inlet nozzle

Air Flow

Sleeve closes preventing backflow of air

Sleeve opens - allows air to escape

Air Flow

A flutter valve, a.k.a. Heimlich valve, is a one-way valve used to prevent air from traveling back into the chest through the chest tube. You can buy one for your kit, or make one if you need.
Photos from ali@sketchymedicine.com

To start we'll need to improvise a decompression needle. You can buy all of this in a pre-packaged kit. Purchased catheters are larger and sturdier than what we'll be using. They also clog less frequently. Something that's always been a problem for the decompression technique. Being preppers though, we'll want to learn how to build one ourselves. What we have planned would make both MacGyver and Mickey Mouse equally proud!

You may remember this image from several chapters back. It's our improvised I.V. needle and catheter.

Making a Decompression Needle

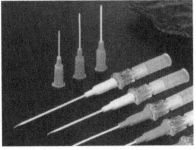
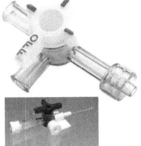

To make a thoracostomy needle for decompressing a pneumo-thorax, find the largest bore I.V. catheter you can. Insert it into the anterior chest wall between the 2nd & 3rd ribs, halfway between the nipple and sternum. Pull the needle out so only the plastic remains. Attach a closed stopcock or syringe. Open the valve every 15 minutes or so to release the air.

You'll insert this 14 or 16 gauge needle into the anterior chest wall, between the 2nd and 3rd, or 3rd and 4th ribs at the "mid-clavicular line." Just find the midpoint of the collar bone (the clavicle) - and feel the rib right under it. This is the second rib. You can insert it here or go down one more.

When inserting the needle between the ribs you've chosen, put it directly above the lower rib, not right underneath the higher one. The blood vessels supplying the ribs run on their inferior surface. So you always insert your catheter right above a rib's upper surface. It's said you always "ride the rib" to prevent puncturing through its blood vessels.

Puncture through the skin, then slowly advance the needle and its plastic covering. After an inch or so in you feel a popping sensation, and air will rush out through the needle.   You're now in the chest cavity.

Advance the plastic catheter overlying the needle another ½ inch.   If the escaping air suddenly stops flowing, you've advanced the plastic catheter too far.   Slowly pull it back, little by little, until airflow returns.   Now it's in perfect position.   It may take several minutes for all of the air to drain from the chest, because your needle and catheter bore size are quite small.

Use this time to tape 4x4 gauze around the needle/catheter to secure it into place.   You'll want to do this now, while you still know it's in perfect position.

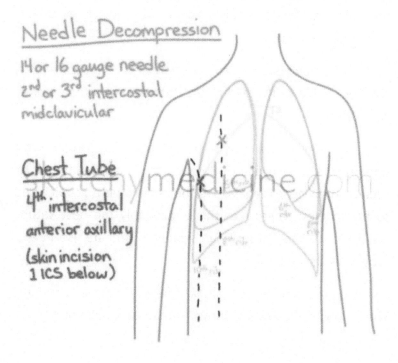

Needle Decompression

14 or 16 gauge needle
2nd or 3rd intercostal
midclavicular

Chest Tube
4th intercostal
anterior axillary
(skin incision
1 ICS below)

Once secured, slowly pull the I.V. needle out of the catheter. Most of the time the walls of the plastic catheter don't collapse into themselves and pinch off. If they do, you'll have to leave the needle partially in, until the "kink" resolves. You'd rather not leave the metal needle inside the catheter unless you have to. The sharp tip can lacerate the lung further if it drifts past its plastic covering and sticks out. (See the picture with the I.V. catheters on the previous page.)

Now that the air has be released, and the chest has been decompressed, the hard part is over. But with the catheter end facing you still open, air can be sucked back through the plastic tubing and reenter the chest cavity. We'll need to fix that.

You have two choices at this point. You can affix a stopcock valve to the end of the catheter, or attach a one-way valve.

If you use a stopcock, release the pressure by opening the valve every 15-30 minutes. Allow all the air to escape, then close it again. If the person has no choice but to be up moving around, this is probably the best setup. We'll call it "the Three Kings system," after its use in the movie discussed earlier.

But it's better to use a one-way valve if you can. The following illustration shows you how to make one:

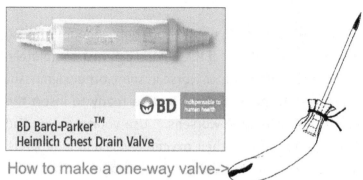

BD Bard-Parker™
Heimlich Chest Drain Valve

How to make a one-way valve->

To improvise a one-way valve, use a condom or cut off the finger of a rubber glove. Then cut a small hole at the end. When the person takes a breath in, the rubber walls will collapse in on themselves, preventing air from the outside from being sucked back into the chest.

Needle decompression is typically used in a pinch. Instances when a person is suspected to have a tension pneumothorax, or has worsening shortness of breath, and needs immediate relief.   The preferred treatment is a chest tube, but that's going to be impractical when the ugly times fall upon us.   Our method works well, and needs to be used if the person has a tension pneumothorax.   I've used it several times myself.   Keep in mind these kink off or become clogged frequently.   Should this occur, you'll need to completely remove it insert a new one.

In the absence of a tension pneumothorax, or continued air leakage from a lacerated lung, the collection will resolve spontaneously without treatment.   But it does so very slowly.   A pokey rate of 1% per day.   This means if 50% of the lung has collapsed, it will take 50 days to fully re-inflate unless you decompress it.   Quite a while!

Our advice about treating a regular pneumothorax, without tension, is this: If the person can rest completely, and is not short of breath or worse in some other significant way, just watch them carefully and be ready to insert the needle if their condition worsens.   Use your pulse ox and stethoscope to monitor their oxygen levels and lung fields. Try to get away with not doing this procedure.   Save it for situations where the person is having difficulty breathing or getting worse.

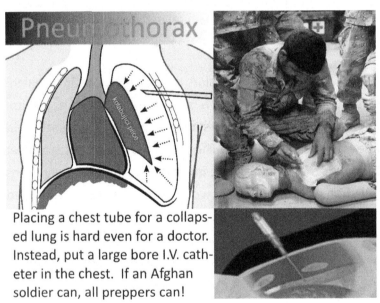

Placing a chest tube for a collapsed lung is hard even for a doctor. Instead, put a large bore I.V. catheter in the chest. If an Afghan soldier can, all preppers can!

At this point, you may be thinking doctors are obsessed with punching holes through people's rib cages. But that's not quite the case.

Let me explain:

Have you ever seen an article or book describing how to take a pocket knife and cut underneath someone's Adam's apple, then shove a straw or broken pen in their trachea so they can breathe?   A sort of last ditch effort for saving someone who's choking and suffocating? We have absolutely no idea why so much emphasis is placed on teaching people that.

The situation is astronomically rare.   But getting shot or impelled through the chest isn't.   Even in normal times, it's an occupational hazard of anyone who makes their living carrying a gun.   Imagine what the risk is going to be like when objects are exploding around you, and a trigger finger is a contagious disease most people have caught. Our assertion still stands: chest trauma has never been a stranger to war.

Now let's see what else can kill us!

TENSION PNEUMOTHORAX & SUCKING OR OPEN CHEST WOUNDS

Gunshot and other puncture wounds cut a path through tissue of the chest wall, creating a conduit through which outside air will inevitably travel. It's the same situation as having a chest tube in a person. Each time the person inhales, outside air will be sucked back inside. An opening like this, not caused by a tube you've placed, is called a sucking chest wound. It's dangerous because it's easier for the air to get pulled in, than it is for it to get back out.

These injuries almost always lead to lung collapse. As the collection is building up, the lung is collapsing down. Soon the vessels draining blood back into the heart may succumb to the building pressure. Kinking off, little by little, the heart may lose its ability to fill with blood, and the person dies of a tension pneumothorax.

You'll want to avoid this.

As you might imagine, treating a sucking chest wound requires decompression of the pneumothorax – then keeping outside air from getting back in. It can be difficult to tell when a penetrating chest wound is sucking in air, so it's safest if you assume they all do.

Begin by sealing the chest wound. Put something plastic over the hole, and tape it down. But don't tape all 4 sides. Seal only three or three-and-a-half sides. By doing that you'll be creating a one-way valve. Yes, the same principles we used before, apply here too. Remember with all chest wall injuries, you'll want to watch for signs and symptoms of tension pneumothorax. Let's review what that might look like:

Signs and symptoms of a tension pneumothorax might include some or all of the following:

1. Absent lung sounds on the affected side.
2. Tympanic sounds in the chest to percussion.
3. Severe shortness of breath.
4. Veins on the person's neck can bulge outward (jugular vein distension).
5. They may have blue lips, neck or fingers (cyanosis).
6. Weak pulse
7. Labored and rapid breathing.
8. Decreased level of consciousness.

They look and feel like they are going to die!

If you suspect a tension pneumothorax, or think one might be building, make sure the one way valve function is working, and that air is getting out of the chest. Or better, remove your plastic seal altogether. If you don't get an immediate rush of air back at you, either open the wound up more, or insert a decompression needle.

If you end up removing a chest seal to relieve a tension pneumothorax, it's best to leave it off. Just let the pressure out so the pressure inside the chest with the outside atmosphere will equalize. This may require opening the wound so it's larger than it was originally.

Making the hole bigger isn't an ideal situation, but it will help equalize the pressure. With a simple pneumothorax, the person probably won't die of shock from a tension pneumothorax. Just watch them carefully, and monitor them constantly with your pulse oximeter.

You can see pulmonary infections and trauma are easier to understand and treat than one might think. Moreover, with just a few inexpensive items, they're common illnesses and injuries you can actually do something about. If you are to save lives, most of the salvaging will come from the chapters you just digested.

Let's transition now to something more common, but thankfully, less lethal:

432

SECTION EIGHT
SETTING UP YOUR TREATMENT FACILITY

SETTING UP TRIAGE & PREVENTING THE SPREAD OF INFECTION

Water, shelter, food – in that order. That's what you should be thinking about as you're traveling to your bug-out-location. I know you already know this. But as the group medic you're always scanning the environment and making plans for building an emergency aid station.

You'll need a place where you can build a makeshift latrine facility - *far* below your water source. I can't tell you the number of times in history this has been overlooked. And it still is. "Ebola" is all we'll say on the subject... *for now*. Just remember that when it rains - often independent of their distance from one another - the water source and latrine can become one. Mixing together they'll cause what would otherwise have been a preventable illness.

Find a natural windbreak and set up your aid station there. You'll want to make improvised beds, and get into the practice of keeping them a few feet off the ground. The best way to do this is by using the same technique you'll use for making stretchers.   Keep an eye out for long straight branches or poles as you travel.   You'll need them to build your stretcher beds.

Now let's find out how to make and set up those beds once you've selected your spot.

KEEPING EBOLA OFF THE BED - CRAFTING DISPOSABLE TRIAGE BEDDING

Take a canvas or one or two bed sheets and stretch them out. Then roll the ends around two long round poles, creating something resembling a stretcher. You might need to connect the poles with rope and place cross beams in-between. That way they'll stay separated as the person sits down and reclines into sleeping position.

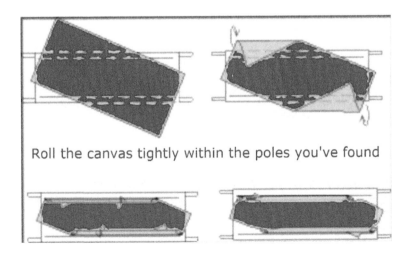

Roll the canvas tightly within the poles you've found

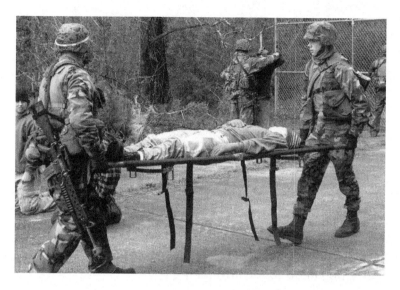

Always use stretchers for beds when you're setting up your aid station. They're not comfortable, *but they are disposable*. That's what you'll need if someone gets Ebola, or one of its friends, on your bedding. If you don't have a canvas or bed sheets, then use shirts or jackets as shown:

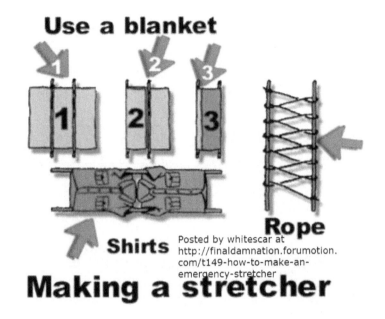

Use a blanket

Rope

Shirts Posted by whitescar at
http://finaldamnation.forumotion.
com/t149-how-to-make-an-
emergency-stretcher

Making a stretcher

Above all, remember these two principles: *keep the stretcher beds off the ground, and sleep people in an alternating head to toe arrangement.*

Keeping beds off the ground prevents unwanted cuddles from rats and snakes attracted to your body heat. Alternating the head-to-toe arrangement is of crucial importance. A lesson the United States Military learned the hard way.

Many infections are spread by respiratory droplets shot into the air when a sick person coughs or sneezes. Many times this occurs even before the person realizes they're getting sick. These microscopic watery spheres, packed with viral particles and sometimes bacteria, travel as far as fifteen feet in the air, where they can remain suspended for hours.

Currently the Centers for Disease Control is sticking to their story that Ebola cannot be transmitted this way. They concede respiratory droplets do carry the virus, but claim there's no evidence people can catch the disease through the air.   Please see our book *The Ebola – American War* for more.

Their official position is that the disease is contagious, meaning it's transmitted by physical contact from one person to another.   But deny it's infectious, meaning it cannot be transmitted via microorganisms in the air or water.

Some of us are skeptical.

The point being that in practice, there's little to no difference in meaning between contagious and infectious when we're talking about a disease or its spread.   The current outbreak of Ebola is unlikely to do much more than alert Americans and Europeans to the likelihood a more dangerous version is on its way.   A sort of wakeup call to those still comatose.

While Ebola is going to be an upcoming and widespread global problem, at present you'll want to be more concerned with other contagious infections like meningitis.   Focus on the diseases that are both contagious and infectious, and can be transmitted at very short distances.   Many don't even require the person be coughing to spread the pathogen. Normal breathing by an infected but seemingly well person can spread the disease.

Early on the military did not know such transmission was possible. And per protocol the beds of soldiers were positioned in a uniform manner; with their heads a cozy two or three feet from one another. Scores of infections tore through barracks for years (not the least of which was meningitis) incapacitating armies and clearing entire battlefields.

In its wake, the military adopted the head-to-toe bed arrangement that's still in use today. They found by increasing the distance between the heads of soldiers 10-15 feet, they were able to reduce communicable airborne diseases to an acceptable level.

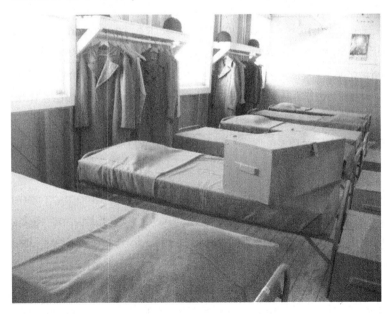

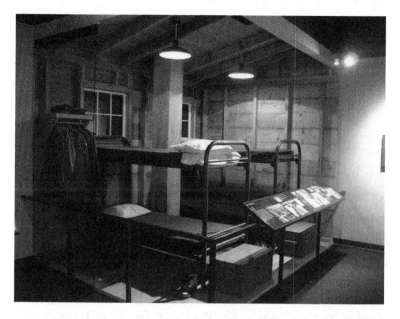

If you've decided to set up in an intact building, especially if it's a small shelter, open opposing windows a bit to encourage air movement outward. Hang plastic semi-transparent plastic sheets - like the tarps used for protecting carpet when painting a room - to isolate the sick as much as possible. By facilitating the movement and outflow of suspended respiratory droplets, your infection rate will drop sharply. It's not a perfect system, but it's likely the best that can be done in austere conditions.

CONTROLLING WHAT CAN'T BE SEEN

If you have members with a contagious infection, start by evaluating its risk of transmission to others. Do this by determining the type of pathogen responsible. Fortunately, in the U.S. and E.U. your options are limited. Parasites for instance, are rare in both places. When they do occur, they're relatively harmless compared to their African and Asian counterparts.

Sure you can get Giardia and a few fungi, but that's often as bad as it gets. For the most part you'll be choosing between a virus and a bacteria as the culprit. And while far from foolproof, there's an easy way to guess which is responsible.

IS IT A VIRUS OR BACTERIA?

Start by counting the number of body areas affected. Viruses generally invade and replicate in as many different sites possible. Not being alive, they must have access to your cellular machinery to replicate – they can't do it on their own. So they hijack and use the cells they're able to gain entry to. In the process they end up destroying tissue in multiple areas.

442

Good old fashion "snot" is a mixture of mucus and the fluid normally found inside your cells. That fluid leaks out as the virus breaks open the cells it's just replicated in, and is leaving to go repeat the processes elsewhere. The carnage claims the lives of millions of cells, housed in tissues ranging from the nose to colon.

Contrast this to bacterial infections. Bacteria prefer to stay put in one area. They set up shop and get established where they land. Only later do they branch out to other areas. That's why a common viral cold gives you a runny nose, sore throat, cough, congestion, stomach upset, and any other number of symptoms. Whereas a bacteria like Strep might cause only tonsillitis. Then later spread to the lungs or sinuses.

Extending this principle, if it's a virus primarily infecting the gastrointestinal system, you'd expect nausea, vomiting, diarrhea, and abdominal pain – evidence that multiple areas of the digestive tract are being injured.

A bacterial infection of the same system might produce vomiting or diarrhea, but is typically limited to one or the other. Only later might it produce symptoms elsewhere. This is not a hard and fast rule, but I think you get the gist of it.

How does all of this help you keep your people from getting sick? Here are the protocols you'll want to teach to your group members:

Mask, Glove and Isolation Protocols

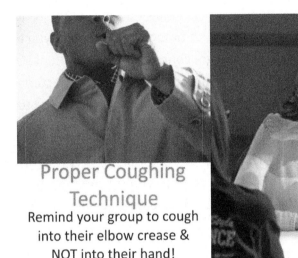

Proper Coughing Technique
Remind your group to cough into their elbow crease & NOT into their hand!

First, remember that regardless if it's viral or bacterial, hand washing and proper coughing technique are always your first countermeasures. Make certain no one is sharing cups or other eating utensils. That said, we recommend the following protocol:

Begin by making an educated guess as to whether the infection is viral or bacterial. If viral, assume it's both airborne and spread by fomites. Encourage your people to wear masks, and separate the ill from the healthy to whatever extent possible.

Viruses you'll be most worried about are typically more infectious than common bacteria. Assume they're airborne, and that the most important fomites are the items containing the food and water supply. Those containers are often the central hub all group members handle.

Charge a well person - one kept away from the sick - with making all the meals and handling the water. *Make sure that person wears gloves and a mask during meal preparation!* Tell them to pretend as if they were the sick one, and everyone else is still healthy. That will help them pay attention to what they're doing, and not stick their finger in the soup and taste it.

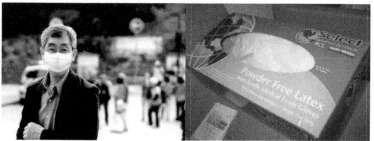

If illness starts spreading through you're camp or BOL, limit infection by assigning 1 person to meal preparation & water. Make them wear a mask & gloves when preparing food!

If you think the illness is bacterial, focus on finding the fomites, and any other item encouraging spread. Remember with both viruses and bacteria, often it's a well appearing person that's the fomite. Masks and isolation may not be as important as limiting personal contact.

It's felt by some that if the person has been taking antibiotics for 24-48 hours, they might have a decreased ability to transmit a bacterial disease. But no one knows for sure.

There are about a million exceptions to the rules I've outlined here. But they'll allow you to develop a plan to deal with what's making your group ill. They're the same guidelines I'll be using in the difficult situations we'll all be facing soon.

We have something really cool to show you next. The amazing 5 gallon bucket!

DISINFECTING LINENS, BEDDING, & CLOTHES – THE AMAZING 5 GALLON BUCKET

Dirty clothes can lead to body lice and ringworm infections. We've discovered this happened frequently to the WWII preppers. Stuck in musty bomb shelters for extended periods of time, and often wearing damp clothing they couldn't change out of, many became susceptible to skin infections. Making things worse, options for treating fungal infections, like ringworm, were very limited at the time.

Dirty bed sheets can also lead to scabies, bedbugs, diseases carried by mouse and rat droppings, and a million other things most of us don't want to think about. As the medic you'll want to be proactive in their prevention. Constructing an improvised field washing machine will help you stay on top of these before they take hold.

All you'll need is a five-gallon bucket with a lid that secures into place, and an unused or extremely well disinfected plunger. Items you can easily scrounge.

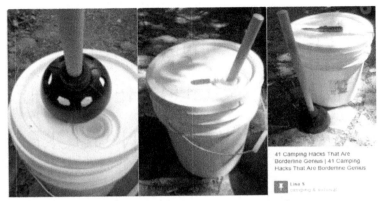

41 Camping Hacks That Are
Borderline Genius | 41 Camping
Hacks That Are Borderline Genius

Lisa S

Making a Chlorine & Soap Disinfection
Washer for Clothing, Bedding & Gear Lisa S - Pintrest

Fill the bucket half full with clean water and add a small amount of bleach.   The bleach won't kill body lice, but it will inhibit the fungus causing ringworm, and help lower viral and bacterial counts.   Equally important, clean clothes and sheets help people feel human again. Something quickly lost in the absence of running water and warm showers.

Next up: Tricks for lighting up your triage!

IMPROVING EFFECTIVE MOOD LIGHTING FOR YOUR TRIAGE

Light discipline can be a tricky subject. At times you'll want to avoid shinning bright beams of light around so as not to give your position away. Yet at the same time you'll need enough illumination to take care of your patients. There's a good solution to this problem. Make a lantern with a head lamp and a milk jug filled with water.

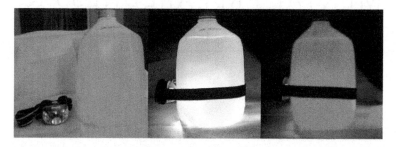

Light discipline can be tricky. Fill a milk jug with water and wrap your headlamp around it to make a lantern. Use white light when you are treating people, then switch to red light if you want to decrease the distance at which it can be seen.

Variations on this theme involve placing a battery powered low level light inside an empty Jiffy Peanut Butter jar, or using a light and some other type of semi-opaque container.

SECTION NINE
MENTAL PREPAREDNESS & FEAR CONTROL

CLUBBING DEPRESSION

Depression is a valuable commodity. It's been bought and sold and used to demoralize troops and countries in every war. Tokyo Rose and Germany's Lord Haw-Haw tried dispensing it over the airwaves in the Second World War. But mostly sucked at it. They knew a person's mental state directly affected their ability to function. So they tried.

Treating depression is almost never a topic in prepper books. But must be addressed. Not only does it impair the person's ability to function, but also that of those around them. People are going to be sad; how could they not after society has collapsed? After their world's been taken away? But sadness and depression are distinctly different entities, and can best be understood in the following way:

SADNESS

Sadness is a normal and healthy emotional reaction to life when things are going poorly. It can last as long as the conditions causing it continue to worsen. Like grief, it should only last about a year, most people acclimate by then. If it doesn't, then sadness and grief turn into depression.

DEPRESSION

Depression can also be thought of as an unhealthy emotional reaction to life. One that occurs even when things are going well. Many of us feel it's poorly understood by modern medicine. And even more poorly treated. This is not for lack of trying. Psychiatry and psychology are both incredibly complex arts and sciences. Their practitioners are usually phenomenal. It's just that the science is still in its infancy. And treating depression as an emergency is limited to hospital admissions and suicide prevention protocols. These remain in place until the episode resolves, medications like Prozac begin to work, or both. In everyday life, this is the best treatment and should be pursued at all costs to ensure the persons safety. But with the types of situations we're talking about, it will have to be treated much differently.

Like all advice I have given in this book, it's only to be used if professional medical care is not, and will not be available. In that case, the following are only my suggestions, for whatever they may be worth.

Selective Serotonin Reuptake Inhibitors, like Prozac and Zoloft, are much safer to take and have fewer side effects than their predecessors. But they take an awfully long time to start working. Two to six weeks is the norm, and even after that the dose must sometimes be increased.

Clearly, this is not going to be a quick fix in emergent situations.

In the olden days, psychiatrists would sometimes give Ritalin to people with major depression. A week or two supply, until the medications of the day like lithium started to take effect. It can be dangerous. But "speed" may be a short term fix for people who have given up. People that would probably lay down die otherwise.

Of course if they are really depressed, and you give them amphetamines, they might just get up the energy they need to kill themselves. Prozac did this. Although it's not a Ritalin like drug, when it first came out it did increase people's energy, and the suicide rate did increased.

Another consideration is addiction. One might see that a perpetual problem could result in a situation like this. Escapes in times of horrific disasters are slam dunks for addictions taking foothold. The saving grace here is that it's going to be very hard to find. So the pills you do get, are likely the only supply you will see for years. That in itself limits potential problems. This brings us to the next controversial emergency treatment... Ketamine.

Believe it or not, this drug is undergoing clinical trials as this book is being written. Ketamine is a club drug. The kids call it "Vitamin K" or "Special K" or Lord knows what. Ketamine seems to reverse profound depression within 30 minutes of taking it, making it an excellent choice for emergency treatment.

I have not been providing references for many of the topics discussed in this book, because some I have offered are out of the realm of conventional medicine. They're tailored specifically for the prepper. In this instance I will. One of the articles about the emergency use of ketamine can be found in: Psychiatric Times (New Claims and Findings for Ketamine in Severe Depression January 17, 2013 | By Arline Kaplan - See more at: http://www.psychiatrictimes.com/major-depressive-disorder/new-claims-and-findings-ketamine-severe-depression#sthash.bILIYaBV.dpuf)

MORE ON PSYCHOLOGICAL PREPAREDNESS

Psychological health is every bit as important as physical health, they are two sides of the same coin. Neither separate from the other.

Every bug-out bag should have in it a deck of cards, and a pair of dice. It should also have a few pieces of hard candy. I learned this from a physician that was pinned in by a storm and stuck in snow cave for nine days. Fortunately he had another person with him to keep him company. But both understandably became quite depressed. They played cards day after day, but even that distraction could only work for so long. Apparently things got quite grim. Both were ready to give up, and just go to sleep... permanently.

Then one of them found a couple of hard mint candies in their bag. He told me that the little bit of sugar made all the difference in their attitude, just when it was most needed.   It was not a grandiose or even entertaining story, but one of those communications where you could feel its importance.   Since that day I have recommend carrying candy and cards on every outdoor trip.

In an apocalypse, expect profound depression.
But also expect profound fear.   Let's tackle that
mammoth next!

HOW TO MANAGE FEAR

Fear has always been a problem for the military, and until recently they weren't quite sure what to do about it. But within the last decade the navy commissioned studies and implemented programs on how to deal with fear. They've decreased their washout rate in the SEAL program by 8% - impressive when you consider it involves overcoming the very real fear of drowning. In this chapter we'll discuss their program, and learn how to implement one of its most effective features into our preps.

There are four techniques to their regime: Goal setting, mental rehearsal, breathing focus, and self-talk.

We'll be discussing the one we should all be addressing daily. It's called negative self-talk, and only recently has the neuroscience behind how it works been discovered.

FEAR IS NOT YOUR FAULT - IT'S DUE TO A GENETIC MISADVENTURE

According to geneticists, about 75,000 years ago humanity underwent a brain upgrade. And like some upgrades do, it went sideways almost immediately. Called "the default mode network," this unique mutation caused humans to start hearing an inner narrative not experienced before by any member of our species. Suddenly people were hearing voices that seemed to be coming out of nowhere.

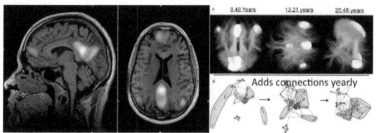

This is what we are up against. Only recently discovered, it's called "The Default Mode Network," and when we are not focused on a task, it kicks in and starts chatting with us at a rate of 300-1000 words per minute. It produces mostly negative self-talk, and is fully developed by age 25!

Anthropologists speculate some early peoples went insane. While others began acting on the new and sometimes homicidal suggestions echoing in their minds. By now modern man has become accustom to this incessant voice, never realizing it's abnormal.

It seems nearly every waking hour we hear our inner voice remind us of what we've done wrong, and what we're going to do wrong. Over, and over, and over. It's relentless. While it shuffles the words around from time to time, the basic message remains the same – "you suck, you always have, and you're going to die!"

The Mechanism is on Autopilot - The Brain is an Organ that Secretes Thoughts in the Same Way the Stomach Secretes Acid

Neuroscientists have counted the rate at which the network speaks - and impressive 300-1000 words a minute. The navy took this seriously, and began teaching candidates to become aware of this automatic self-slaughter - and to take action!

At this level of military training no one is a "boot camp maggot" any longer. This situation is for 'reals' as they say, and young warriors now practice identifying and replacing negative dialog with positive and encouraging inner chatter. They report it takes time, after all it involves breaking a lifelong and genetically driven habit. But it's a perfect place for preppers to start, and may come easier to them as they're already in the habit of preparing themselves.

It's important to know how to make children, and even adults, feel better when they're sick. That's up next!

FEELING BETTER WHEN YOU'RE SICK

When we're ill we take for granted the safety and warmth our homes, and forget that one day it might all disappear. And so we've forgotten the simple things we can do to comfort ourselves and our children in times of sickness.

Helping Children Feel Better When Sick

- Radiant and evaporative heat loss occur with fever, and are more pronounced in children. Keep them warm with layered clothing and blankets.
- Give warm fluids and food.
- Water is needed for metabolism, being ill increases metabolism so give the child as much fluid as they can take in.
- Have them cuddle with a pet. It's unlikely that one will be available in a disaster, but you can make them a stuffed animal with a sock and some buttons.
- Comfort foods and music help if available.

Helping Adults Feel Better When Sick

- o Take a couple of showers a day if warm water is available.
- o Stay warm with layered clothing and blankets.
- o Sit out in the sun if you can twice daily.
- o Take frequent naps.
- o Stretch twice daily for as long as possible, this releases endorphins.
- o Warm fluids and comfort foods, just as you would with a child.
- o Zone out on Benadryl and perform saline nasal washings if stuffy

Our Sincere Thanks to All of You!

We hope you'll never have to use any of the information presented in this book. Writing something like this is consider fear mongering in the medical profession. But knowing what to do if anything like this were to happen, helps alleviate fear. That's why it's been written. Preparing is often the only recourse we have in our rapidly changing and unpredictable world.

We hope you have enjoyed this book. Before visiting our appendix for additional information on suturing and other surgical skills, please leave us a review, we could sure use a lot of them!

Finally, thanks to all you that have been following us at ThePrepperPages.com, and have suggested topics for discussion. If you have any medical questions you'd like answered, please leave us a note and we'll look into it!

Without reviews on Amazon, independent home grown books like this one quickly wither away and die! So if you have a moment, please leave us a review and tell us what you liked about this guide. If you have any suggestions for future books that might serve the prepper community, please let us know. We only write on medical issues, for all other prepping tips, we buy and read your books! If you have one, and would like it reviewed, leave us a note on our site and we'll get right to it! Thanks again!

ABOUT THE AUTHOR

Dr. Chamberlin is a surgeon and medical professor specializing in neuroscience, medical genomics, clinical pathology, and anatomy. He writes narrative medicine (creative non-fiction) 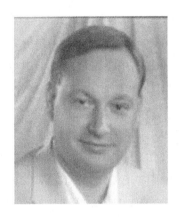 and can be contacted at: doctorryanc@gmail.com or through ThePrepperPages.com website, for inquires, comments or questions.

APPENDICES

Appendix A – Things to Collect

GARAGE

- DUCT TAPE
- BOX CUTTER
- STIFF WIRE
- LIGHTERS
- FISHING LINE
- NEEDLE NOSE PLIERS
- SYNRINGES & NEEDLES
- HAND SANITIZER
- INNER TUBE OR SURGICAL TUBING
- HEAD LAMP FLASHLIGHT
- HAND BUTANE TORCH

KITCHEN

- BLACK TRASH BAGS
- ZIPLOCK BAGS
- COFFEE FILTERS
- SPONGE
- DISH WASHING GLOVES
- SEWING KIT
- SPRAY BOTTLE
- LIGHTERS
- SMALL METAL THERMOS
- HONEY

LINEN CLOSET & FAMILY ROOM

- PLAIN WHITE PILLOW CASES
- X-ACTO
- BATTERIES
- FLASH LIGHT

BATHROOM

- BAR SOAP
- VASOLENE
- COTTON BALLS
- TWEEZERS
- MEDICATIONS
- RUBBING ALCOHOL
- ANY MEDICAL SUPPLIES
- HAND SANITIZERS

MEDICAL OFFICES

- MPR
- TONGUE DEPRESSORS
- SUPPLIES HIDDEN UNDER DESK

PHARMACY, STORE & PET SHOP

- BETADINE AND ANTISEPTICS
- DROPPER BOTTLE
- VITAMINS
- ELECTROLYTE MIXES
- FISH

KID'S ROOMS

- X-ACTO
- FISH ANTIBIOTICS
- HEADLAMP
- HERBALS

LAUNDRY ROOM

- BLEACH
- BAR SOAP
- SPRAY BOTTLE

Appendix B - Tying Suture

SQUARE KNOT

Start the practice of suturing with the most basic of knots: the "Square knot."   This style is used in *all* suturing to tie any type of material being used.   It's easy to perform and can be done quickly.   Practice the "Surgeon's knot" often. To do this, tie a knot like you usually would, but loop the thread under twice, not once like you typically would.   Use this technique on the first throw only; it helps keep the knot from slipping, as you reconnoiter and tie the second.

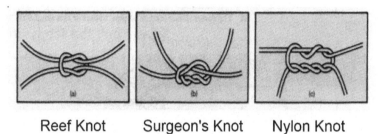

Reef Knot   Surgeon's Knot   Nylon Knot

INSTRUMENT TYING WITH A PIG'S FOOT

Refer to this section for step-by-step instructions on basic suturing technique.   Use pigs' feet or chicken drumsticks.

1.   Using a practice incision, insert the needle about 1/8 - 1/4 in. from the edge, penetrate the full thickness of the skin and bring the needle out the other side about the same distance back from the edge, leaving about 4 - 5 cm (1.5 - 2.0 in.) on the short end of the suture.

2. Take up slack with the needle end (long end) of the suture in the palm of your hand.

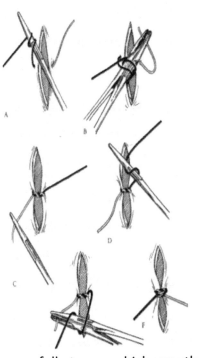

3. Bringing the needle holder across the wound from the short end to the long end of the suture, loop the suture twice around the tip of the needle holder (Figure A).

4. Open the needle holder, grasp the short end of the suture, and gently pull the loops off the needle holder and reverse your hands (Figures B and C).

5. Stop! Look carefully to see which way the double loop will lay most evenly and pull most snugly. This knot should be slightly looser than the ultimate tension desired on the wound, as the second knot will slightly tighten the tie.

6. If necessary, reverse the short and long ends of the suture to lock the first stitch.

7. Bring the needle holder across the wound f the short end into the long end of the suture, make a single loop (Figure D), and again grasp the short end (Figure E), pull the loop off the needle holder, and reverse your hands (Figure F).

8.   Carefully look to make sure the knot is even and square to the first knot before tightening.

9.   Repeat steps 7 and 8.

Supplies Needed for Suture Practice

o   **Drapes**: These can be disposable, packaged, surgical drapes or sterile packaged towels.
o   **Suture**: 6-0 nylon for face; 5-0 and 4-0 where stronger suture is required; 5-0 and 4-0 Vicryl for deep suture, because they will   dissolve. Polyglactin will dissolve faster than Vicryl.
o   **Anesthetic**: 1% lidocaine, with or without epinephrine, and 0.25% bupivacaine.
o   **Antibacterial cleaning agents**: Povidone-iodine (Betadine) or whatever you'll be using in the field.
o   **Syringes and needles**: 3-to 5-mL syringe for local anesthetic, 30 to 60mL syringe for irrigation; 20-22 gauge needle for drawing up anesthetic and 18-20 for irrigation, 25-gauge or smaller needle for local infiltration.
o   **Irrigation solution**: 1 L normal saline (0.9%).
o   **Sharps container**: For needles and suture needles.
o   **Dressings**: Non-adherent dressings, gauze sponges and hypoallergenic tape.

Appendix C - Simple Interrupted Suture Technique

The simple interrupted stitch is the most fundamental and common stitch used in laceration repair. It can anchor a wide wound well, evert the edges of a narrow wound, and precisely close a wound with edges of different height.

When this stitch is properly performed, the flask shape of the needle and suture path will gently and evenly evert the edges of the wound (Figures B and C.) When the stitch is performed incorrectly, the wound edges are inverted rather than everted, as shown in Figure A. Inverted wound closure results in scars that are more noticeable, particularly in tangential light. Wounds with one edge higher than the other can be closed by varying the depth of the suture, so that it's shallow on high side, and deeper on low side (Fig. F). The length of the wound that is closed by one stitch will vary by the size of the bite, and distance from the needle pass to the incision (Figure D). You can see how the larger the bite, the greater the wound length closed with each stitch.

Disadvantages of the simple interrupted stitch include "railroad track" scarring, occasional inversion of the wound edges, and the fact that it's time consuming.

The first two of these disadvantages can be minimized by careful placement of sutures. Specifically by making sure wound edges are everted and equal on both sides. The proper tension is also important. A stitch that's too tight can cause puckering and accentuate railroad tracks. You want to gently "kiss" the everted wound edges. In general surgery we say "approximation without strangulation." Proper timing of suture removal is essential. Left in too long, and scar tissue will begin to form around the suture material.

1)   For most wounds, beginning to stitch in the middle of the wound and following the rule of halves provides even closure.

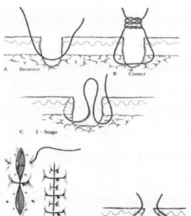

2)   Place the needle in the needle holder and begin your stitch with the needle tip pointing perpendicular to the skin. The needle should be held in the tip of the needle holder, about one-third of the way down on the needle curve. This gives the best control and prevents the needle from bending.

3)   Going through both sides of the wound in one motion is best, exiting the skin directly opposite and at the same distance from the wound margin as the entrance (Figure D).

4)   But if the bite required will be too big, the stitch can be done in two motions, as shown in Figure C.

5)   By using your finger or forceps, you can help the needle exit less traumatically, but can also cause you to accidently stick yourself.   ALWAYS GRAB THE NEEDLE WITH YOUR NEEDLE DRIVER TO PULL IT OUT ON THE EMERGING SIDE!!!

6)   Tie with an instrument tie or with a square knot by hand.

7)   When done correctly, the flask-shaped path of the suture, and proper tension on the knot, should result in an everted wound edge.   This is important, because as the wound heals, the scar pulls away from the cut, and the everted edge flattens as it heals like you want.

8)   Repeat the procedure until the wound is closed, varying the size of the bite (distance from the suture line) a little each time. This prevents the wound from tearing under stress, like old perforated postage stamps used to.   Remember that a wider bite closes a larger length of the wound than a smaller bite.

Appendix D - Running Sutures

Running sutures belong to a group of stitches that start at the end of a laceration and run the whole length, ending up opposite from where it started. There are two basic running stitches: basic running and running locking.

Both are convenient and rapid means of suturing well-approximated wound edges on which little tension is placed. They are used on the neck, scrotum, or wherever loose skin is found. They should not be used if the wound requires deeply placed stitches, or where dead space has not previously been closed.

When practicing with a pig's foot, make a two or three inch narrow excision in the skin. Then proceed through the

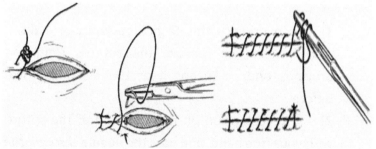

following steps:

    1) *In any running suture you begin at the wound end that is farthest from you,* put a suture in and tie it, and then cut the short end *only*.

2)   Always sew towards yourself!

3)   Make evenly placed interrupted passes with the needle as you travel down the entire length of the wound.

4)   With the last stitch, leave a loose "loop" and use it to tie the suture.   There are only two knots in a running suture: the one that anchors it in the beginning, and the one that completes it when the end has been reached.

5)   When working with this loop of suture, the one you've left upon the sutures completion, grasp it with one hand, and the needle end with the other.

6)   Tie several square knots and cut both ends.

Running and Locking Sutures

1)   To practice this technique you can make a new incision, or remove the sutures from the previous one.   Anchor it at the distal end like before.

2)   Keep tension on the long end of the suture with your free hand, and pass the needle *through the loop* before making the next stitch.

3)   To do this, watch the needle tip as it exits the skin, then make a loop in the suture with your free hand.

4)   Pass the needle-holder tip through this loop, grasp the needle point, and pull through the loop creating a "locked" stitch.

5)   Repeat steps 2 and 3 for the length of the wound.

6)   Place your last stitch without the lock, so as to leave a looped end with which to tie.

7)   Tie off as usual.

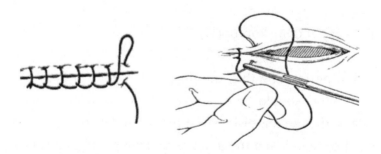

Appendix E – Vertical Mattress Sutures

You may choose to use the vertical mattress stitch in certain circumstances. Properly placed, it everts the edges better others. It can be chosen when you need to close large area of dead space in a wound. It's a strong stitch providing some added support to a wound under stress. Perhaps its most common role is to provide a "stay" suture to initially approximate and align a wound to be closed using other types of stitches.

Disadvantages of the vertical mattress stitch is that placement is time consuming, especially when care is taken to perform it properly. Also, it can result in "railroad tracking" if done improperly.

When performing this, the deep stitch goes in first. The first "bite" should be of equal distance from both wound edges; though this distance varies depending on the tension on the wound, and the amount of dead space to be closed. Generally this will be about ¼ inch back from the edge.

The second bite is much shorter, and should also be of equal distances from the wound edges. This equates to about 1/16 inch from the edge, and serves to provide the even eversion your trying to create.

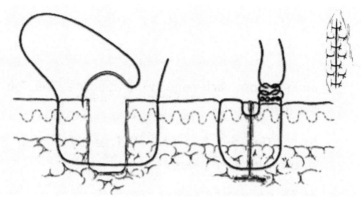

Next, pull the edges of the wound gently and evenly together to provide equal tissue approximation at all levels of the wound. Remember to use equal tension on each stitch.

1)   The amount of tension on the wound will determine the distance from the edges your first and deep bite should go. The more tension, the deeper the bite will need to be.

2)   Begin in the middle of the wound with the rule of halves.

3)   With the needle pointing perpendicular to the skin, make the first deep bite on both sides of the wound equidistant from the wound edges.   Make the bite at least ¼ inch from the edge.   If the bite needed is very large, come out in the middle of the wound and re-grasp the needle to finish the stitch.

4)   Now you will need to shorten the curve.   Do this by grasping the needle in the middle, and placing a shallow interrupted stitch approximately 1/16th of

an inch from each edge in the opposite direction of the first pass.

5)   Tie your first knot and gently tighten the suture with even pressure.

6)   Place your next two knots squarely.

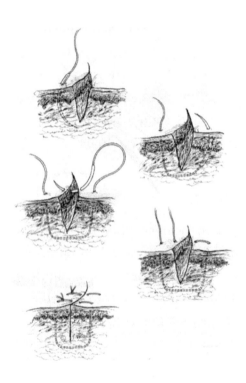

Appendix F – Buried Sutures

Buried sutures are used for providing wound stability and closing dead space.   It can also help evert the skin edges and relieve excessive tension on the wound.

Remember not to pull the stitch too tightly or tissue necrosis (cell death) may result.   Stick to the surgical mantra "approximation without strangulation."

Choose where you anchor the stitch carefully. Placing a stitch only in fat, will cause it to pull through when it is tied or stress.   Avoid this by including a portion of the deep skin or tissue covering (called fascia) with each deep suture. The major purpose of this stitch is to close dead space, so you must make sure your final product is deep enough.

The knot is buried in this stitch. Instrument ties can be difficult in deep wounds where traction near the knot is needed to pull the tissue together.   When tying the knot, pull parallel to the axis of the wound.   This will help get the best tissue approximation possible.

How you position the knot is important. In very deep wounds, the knot can be positioned upward without causing a bump or tissue reaction (Figures A and C). However, in the wounds you will be making on the pigs' feet, the subcutaneous stitch will be more superficial and the knot should be buried (Figures B and D).

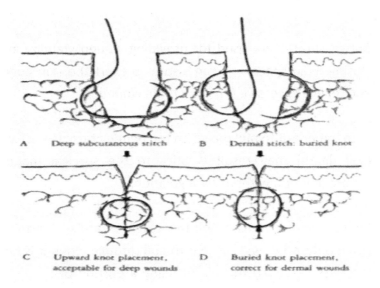

A   Deep subcutaneous stitch   B   Dermal stitch: buried knot

C   Upward knot placement,   D   Buried knot placement,
    acceptable for deep wounds   correct for dermal wounds

1)   The position of the knot, whether it ends up on top or on bottom, will depend on the direction of the first bite. For instance in figure A, the needle is pointed down with first bite, causing the knot to appear on top.   However in figure B, the needle is pointed up with the first bite, so the knot is formed underneath or "buried."

2)   The rest of the mechanics of this stitch are the same as those of the simple interrupted stitch.

3)   Close the wound by alternating knots up and down while making sure your stitch is deep enough.

4)   It's best to practice both hand and instrument ties to see which is easiest for you.

5)   Close the top layer of the wound with any stitch you want.

Appendix G – Undermining & Debridement

Before closing the wound, devitalized tissue must be cut away, or debrided.   Debridement and wound cleaning are the two most important steps and must be done before the wound is closed.

If the wound edges cannot be easily approximated, they may need to be undermined so the skin can be brought together without tension.   Undermining is done by carefully dissecting the outer layer of skin from its dermal attachment, thereby achieving decreased skin tension. When the wound is deep, use an absorbable deep suture like Vicryl.   This will eliminate dead space, which left alone could provide a site for hematoma or abscess.   When the edges are uneven or jagged, clean them up by trimming the uneven tissue with scalpel or scissors

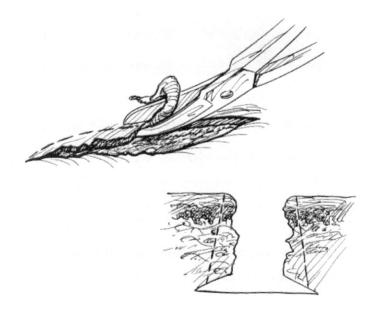

When a portion of the skin is removed by trauma or debridement, a hole is left in the skin.   Then when you try to close it by pulling it together, there's tension on the incision line, which will cause the wound spring apart. Over time, this tension will cause the resultant scar to spread and increase in size.   More importantly, excess tension will make the repair fall apart, and the wound will reopen when you least want it to.

Undermining can be accomplished with a surgical blade or sharp scissors, or by blunt dissection with scissors.

Blunt dissection is preferred because the underlying tissues will tear harmlessly around the blood vessels and nerves. This is in contrast to sharp dissection, which does cut nerves and blood vessels, and results in added trauma and bleeding.

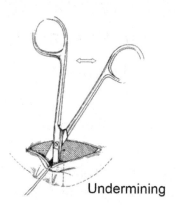

Undermining

There is no hard and fast rule for how far from the incision line you should undermine. Factors like the location on the body, and the elasticity of the skin in the injured area, play important roles in the determination. A helpful rule is to undermine each side the length of the incision. Then if the tension persists on the wound edge, undermine it further before suturing it closed.

Appendix H – Wound Care - What to do When the Laceration is Healing

The wound area should be kept dry and inspected every day by the person for signs of infection. Redness, swelling, warmth, tenderness, or drainage are all indicators that this has occurred, and that the wound might need to be re-opened and drained.

Many people will put antibiotic ointment over the wound for the first several days, though it's uncertain if it is helpful.

Most of the time stitches, or staples, should be removed three to five days after repair of facial lacerations. Seven to eight days after closure of a scalp or extremity wound. And 10 to 14 days following the stitching of wounds over mobile joints and on the soles, palms, or back.

Appendix I – Removing Sutures

Sometimes sutures can be very difficult to remove, especially when they have been left in for several days.

First cut the suture and then pull the knot across the suture line as seen in figure A.   This pulls the suture out in the direction in which it was placed, and avoids putting unwanted tension opposite the axis of the closed wound edge. If the suture is pulled out away from the closure line, wound dehiscence may result (Figure B).

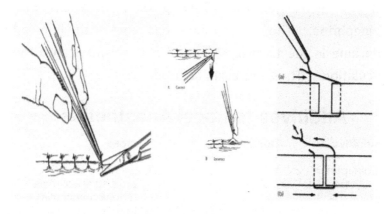

1.   Remove the interrupted stitches placed by cutting the suture and then pulling the knot and suture across the axis of the closed wound.   Can cut the suture material with a scalpel as well.

2.   When removing sutures in the remaining exercises, always use this technique. Be sure to practice it correctly.

Appendix J – Additives to Local Anesthetics - Decreasing the Pain of Injection

Epinephrine and sodium bicarbonate are both common additives to local anesthetics. In the case of epinephrine, the additive is mixed with the lidocaine at the factory, and comes in a bottle with a red label as we discussed before. Epinephrine helps decrease bleeding from wound edges, and you can use more of it than plain lidocaine. 4 ml/kg for 1% plain lidocaine, versus 7mg/kg for 1% lidocaine with epinephrine. The epinephrine keeps more of the injected lidocaine in the tissues, so less of it is absorbed into the circulation. Thus, more can be used.

Additives to Local Anesthetics

Additive	Dosage	Purpose
Epinephrine (adrenaline)	1 : 100 000 or less	To decrease bleeding, prolong anesthesia, reduce anesthetic toxicity
Sodium bicarbonate (8.5%)	1 mL (1 mEq/mL) for every 10 mL of 1% lidocaine with epinephrine (adrenaline)	To decrease pain with infiltration of acidic solution

Sodium bicarbonate is sometimes added by the physician to lidocaine without epinephrine. It helps decreases the amount of stinging produced when injected. It's never mixed in the multi-dose vial. Instead, you'll want to mix it in the syringe containing plain lidocaine.   Do this right before you're ready to inject.   The proportions are 1ml of sodium bicarbonate to 9 ml of lidocaine.

Appendix K - Directions for Using an Inhaler

Using an inhaler seems simple, but most patients do not use it the right way. When you use your inhaler the wrong way, less medicine gets to your lungs.

For the next few days, read these steps aloud as you do them or ask someone to read them to you. Ask your doctor or nurse to check how well you are using your inhaler.

Use your inhaler in one of the three ways pictured below. A or B are best, but C can be used if you have trouble with A and B. Your doctor may give you other types of inhalers.

Steps for using your inhaler

Getting ready	1. Take off the cap and shake the inhaler.
	2. Breathe out all the way.
	3. Hold your inhaler the way your doctor said (A, B, or C below).
Breathe in slowly	4. As you start breathing in slowly through your mouth, press down on the inhaler one time. (If you use a holding chamber, first press down on the inhaler. Within 5 seconds, begin to breathe in slowly.)
	5. Keep breathing in slowly, as deeply as you can.
Hold your breath	6. Hold your breath as you count to 10 slowly, if you can.
	7. For inhaled quick-relief medicine (beta$_2$-agonists), wait about 15-30 seconds between puffs. There is no need to wait between puffs for other medicines.

A. Hold inhaler 1 to 2 inches in front of your mouth (about the width of two fingers).

B. Use a spacer/holding chamber. These come in many shapes and can be useful to any patient.

C. Put the inhaler in your mouth. Do not use for steroids.

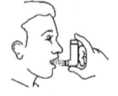 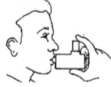 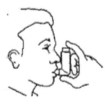

Clean your inhaler as needed, and know when to replace your inhaler. For instructions, read the package insert or talk to your doctor, other health care provider, or pharmacist.

REFERENCES

Quinn J, Wells G, Sutcliffe T, et al: A randomized trial comparing octylcyanoacrylate tissue adhesive and sutures in the management of lacerations. JAMA 1997;277(19):1527-1530

Fraser JJ: Nonfatal injuries in adolescents: United States, 1988. J Adolesc Health 1996;19(3):166-170

Pfeiffer RP, Kronisch RL: Off-road cycling injuries. Sports Med 1995;19(5):311-325

Porras-Reyes BH, Mustoe TA: Wound healing, in Cohen M (ed): Mastery of Plastic and Reconstructive Surgery, ed 1. Boston, Little, Brown and Co, 1994, vol 1

Weinzweig N, Weinzweig J: Basic principles and techniques in plastic surgery, in Cohen M (ed): Mastery of Plastic and Reconstructive Surgery, ed 1. Boston, Little, Brown and Co, 1994, vol 1

Hunt TK, Mueller RV: Wound healing, in Way LW (ed): Current Surgical Diagnosis and Treatment, ed 10. Norwalk, CT, Appleton and Lange, 1994

Dery W: Wound dressing, in Pfenninger JL, Fowler GC (eds): Procedures for Primary Care Physicians, St Louis, Mosby, 1994

Rohrich RJ: Wound healing and closure/abnormal scars/envenomation and extravasation injuries. Selected Readings Plastic Surg 1990;6(1):16-18

Osmond MH, Klassen TP, Quinn JV: Economic comparison of a tissue adhesive and suturing in the repair of pediatric facial lacerations. J Pediatr 1995;126(6):892-895

Bruns TB, Simon HK, McLario DJ, et al: Laceration repair using a tissue adhesive in a children's emergency department. Pediatr 1996;98(4 pt 1):673-675

Rubin, A: Managing Abrasions and Lacerations, The Physician and Sports Medicine May 1998:26(5)

Trott, A, Wounds and Lacerations: Emergency Care and Closure, Second Edition, Mosby, 1997.

Made in the USA
Middletown, DE
21 September 2023